# Dilemmas and Decision Making in Residential Childcare

# Dilemmas and Decision Making in Residential Childcare

**Abbi Jackson**

Routledge
Taylor & Francis Group

LONDON AND NEW YORK

First published in 2023 by Critical Publishing Ltd.

Published 2025 by Routledge
4 Park Square, Milton Park, Abingdon, Oxon OX14 4RN
605 Third Avenue, New York, NY 10017

*Routledge is an imprint of the Taylor & Francis Group, an informa business*

British Library Cataloguing in Publication Data
A CIP record for this book is available from the British Library

ISBN: 9781915080806 (pbk)
ISBN: 9781041055136 (ebk)

Cover and text design by Out of House Ltd

DOI: 10.4324/9781041055136

# CONTENTS

# MEET THE AUTHOR

**Abbi Jackson** has worked in children's services for around 27 years. She has been a foster carer and worked in secure care and children's residential care. She has spent time as a social worker in a statutory childcare team, as an Independent Form F assessor and as a supervising social worker. She has led large-scale practice audits in children and adult services. Currently she is leading quality improvement work in adult social work and integrated services and is an independent panel member for a private fostering company. She offers professional business coaching, inclusive of all career levels.

Abbi is also a very active practice educator and lectures in critical social work practice. She has an interest in early intervention with young people who experience emerging mental health concerns. Never a dull moment, she is currently undertaking a piece of action research with young people in residential care receiving alternative therapies. She is a beekeeper in her spare time.

## Author's note

Please note that the material in this book has been developed from the thoughts of the author as an individual and is not endorsed by any employer, past or present. The examples are fictitious.

# INTRODUCTION

Welcome to this book of ideas. If you are starting out as a new residential childcare worker, or if you are very experienced, I hope you can engage with the fictional case studies in the following pages, to reflect, and help others reflect, on what matters day to day to the children we care for.

There is no other job that brings people together in such a way where we must rely so intensively on our co-workers to care for children who each present with a unique set of needs. Successful practice relies upon accurate communication in a complex environment which is always operating at the edge of chaos. Our personal values and biases play out in real time and our self-regulation is tested over and over. Residential childcare brings out the best and the worst of us all, often both on the same day! Yet, it could be argued that it is a privilege to be afforded the opportunity to use ourselves and our skills to enter into relationships that help children grow.

Children and young people who are placed in residential care provision are likely to have had a range of adverse experiences: complex loss, perhaps bereavement or abandonment, maybe intergenerational poverty, neglect, abuse, and possibly been subject to varying degrees of coercive control and complex relational issues. For whatever reason, they are likely not to have received the type of care that has met their needs fully. They may present with difficulties in attachment and/or they may hold an understanding of their own life story which has been socially constructed around them in unhelpful and confusing ways. In short, their social learning has been challenged and multiple aspects of their development have been impacted.

That said, children and young people in residential childcare are exceptionally resilient and have navigated their difficulties so far. However, we need to bear in mind that this resilience may have led to the young person behaving in certain ways in their family and culture to survive. In their world, this behaviour is perhaps quite rational, functional and adaptive. Yet this same presentation may be considered 'challenging behaviour' in a residential childcare setting, with its rules, boundaries and different social norms.

Knowing each child really matters. Professional curiosity in this instance, however, may not mean that we need to know all (or any) details about their background and life experiences. Although this detail can help us in our approach, it is often inaccessible to workers and sometimes obscured to the young person themselves, albeit they carry the weight in other ways. While we don't need to know why a child behaves in the way they do, we can use good observation skills and tentatively use 'mentalisation' to anticipate their mind states and try our best to attune to their emotional needs (see overleaf).

## Notes

Mentalisation is something we use all the time within our relationships in the widest sense. Examples include the following.

- A friend shares some bad news. We respond in a way that takes account of how we perceive they might be feeling.
- A family member asks for help with a decision, and we think about what might be on their mind before we consider how to frame our comments.

Professional curiosity may mean that we gradually find out what works for this individual young person; what they need and prefer from adults to help them self-regulate. How they tolerate, accept or seek a therapeutic relational distance is important (*so, how much is too much care and, conversely, how much nurture are we willing to give? What does this feel like for both parties?*). We also need to attempt to think about the young person's world through the lens of trauma.

Day to day, the words 'trauma-informed care' are often used in linear or surface-level terms: for example, we know about an aspect of the child's background, so we work in ways to minimise triggering or retraumatising. This sounds sensible and kind; however, 'trauma-informed' in this sense may only be the tip of the iceberg, and somewhat incongruent with the young person's whole lived reality. Given that the trauma many children have experienced may have been when they were pre-verbal, and in the context of relationships during their early years, we may never know what might trigger or destabilise them.

So, how can we practise in a truly trauma-informed way? The only person that can confirm if our responses are trauma informed is the person on the receiving end of our practice. And, even then, they may not be able to articulate why and how this felt 'okay' or 'not okay'. When reflecting on trauma-informed or trauma-sensitive actions, we can ask directly for affirmation of how our practice is felt and perceived. We can ask observers for their comments, or just appreciate and accept the nuances of the unspoken communication instead and continue reflecting. Our best practice then needs to aim for overall *trauma-sensitive care*, where we approach every young person with honesty, integrity, reliability, authenticity, respect and compassion. Especially on the hardest days.

With this as a baseline, this book aims to look at some approaches that residential childcare workers may think about using in practice. It gives examples of why some strategies might be used and the decision making of the fictional worker. All the examples are based on an understanding of how the impact of trauma presents as flight, fight, freeze or fawn responses to stress.

## Extending knowledge

*Dilemmas and Decision Making in Residential Care* should be read alongside texts that explain the nervous system response to trauma in depth along with the science of how co-regulation works.

For example:

- *Why Love Matters: How Affection Shapes a Baby's Brain* by Sue Gerhardt (2014).

- *How to Rewire Your Anxious Brain* by Catherine M Pittman and Elizabeth M Karle (2015).

- *The Pocket Guide to Polyvagal Theory: Transformative Power of Feeling Safe* by Steven Porges (2017).

- *The Neuroscience of Stress, Trauma and Brain Development* by Carol Scherbring (2021).

- *Working with Relational and Developmental Trauma in Children and Adolescents* by Karen Treisman (2016).

- *The Body Keeps the Score: Mind, Brain and Body within the Treatment of Trauma* by Bessel Van Der Kolk (2015).

This book is designed to spark debate and critical thinking among colleagues. It is at first easier to think about practice after it has happened. Teams can give attention to debrief after critical incidents or to more subtle elements of practice to help each other reflect. A culture of improvement and learning could begin with team members verbalising something that went well, and then something that would be *'even better if...'*. This only works when judgement of each other's perceived values and practice is suspended. Reflecting in action often comes later in practice and is only possible when workers' brains are operating in a calm way, with the rational, frontal part of the brain engaged. Neuroscience will quickly tell us that young people need adults who are not stressed and operating principally from the 'feelings' part of the brain. So, it is to everyone's advantage to work on creating a calming, psychologically safe environment.

Thankfully, evidence-based practice can offer a way of helping workers decide what to do: this includes observation, listening, policy, legislation and theory, alongside practice wisdom. This book aims to suggest and use a range of theories to support the development of confident, reflective workers who can think through and apply reasoned judgements. This will help when decisions need to be made and changed quickly in a rapid-paced human system, where a number of people's competing needs must be met simultaneously and compromises are an essential part of group living.

As these challenges are so fundamental to the work in residential care, the case studies in this book can also be used in developing interview formats so that potential candidates can evidence their decision-making competencies for working with multiple children in an unpredictable environment.

The interviewees' ability to assess risk and think on their feet could be measured, as well as their values, potential parenting styles and how they might work alongside others. In supervision, the case studies can be used to tease out themes and to promote agency policy or areas for group practice improvement.

The interventions are not intended to be perfect examples of interactions, so supervisors might highlight what their own expectations are of workers, how the dilemmas raised apply to their unique service provision, and what other options workers might have. There could be wider themes like autonomy, children's rights or relationship-based practice covered in discussion sessions based on the material in this book. Practice educators and trainers can adapt material to suit the specific learning needs of individuals. Flip to the end of the book to find an outline of some theories that could be considered to inform everyday interactions with children and young people. Students might use the learning to support written practice accounts to evidence competencies. Please use the book in any way that fits for you.

You will notice, though, that the stories have some common elements within the fictional workers' responses:

• self-awareness;

• listening;

• considering what behaviour may be communicating;

• validating the person's feelings;*

• validating the person's experiences;*

• validating the person;*

• recognising the person's core strengths;

• offering positive affirmation of the young person's values, attributes, strengths and efforts;

• being predictable to co-regulate;

• doing what they say they will do;

• collaborating with others.

* When validating something, all that needs to be said is 'It looks like...', 'It seems like...' or 'It sounds like...' followed by what you are observing, rather than saying that you 'understand' (which is not possible as you are not party to the subjective or internal experiences of anyone else). This validating language gives the option for the other person to agree or disagree. You can ask them if you are right or wrong. If you are right, the person gains a sense that you are alongside them emotionally. If you are wrong, they can clarify, you can validate again, and both land with a sense of emotional connection. To feel seen and heard is something denied to many children so if you only take one thing from this book, let it be this.

# Lastly, a note about self-care

Residential care work is demanding. By the nature of the role, we bring our whole self to work. The emotional labour is taxing and often seems relentless. Self-care and meeting our own basic needs are essential rather than desirable but are often overlooked as we also try to survive in the complex environment. The fun parts of self-care might be self-explanatory. The less fun parts of self-care need our attention too. For example:

• having difficult conversations;

• doing what you don't feel like doing in the present moment to benefit the future you;

• holding physical and psychological boundaries;

• letting go of habits and choices that are familiar but no longer serve you;

• acknowledging how things are impacting you (and figuring out how to make changes);

• being honest with yourself, especially when the truth is hard to admit;

• being kind to yourself when you get things wrong;

• figuring out who is responsible for what;

• neglecting yourself to take care of someone else may seem like an act of love but giving from a place of emptiness only leads to resentment towards the other person and eventually towards yourself;

• accept that you will disappoint some people when you prioritise your self-care.

> *'If your compassion does not include yourself, it is incomplete.'*
> **Dalai Lama**

# COMMUNICATION MICRO-SKILLS: SELF-REFLECTION

The tool below is designed to be used by anyone in any role. In residential childcare, communication is key in every situation and can be worked on and improved by individuals and groups willing to give attention to detail. This grid can be reproduced for use alone or in supervision and can be revisited periodically. It specifically prompts qualitative reflection and purposely does not include a numerical rating scale; thinking about practice is more important than deciding upon a number to rank skills. Take some time to step back from the pace of practice and decide where you use these skills – think of the subtle examples where these are working well. Then think of where you see the need for improvement and consider how you intend to do things differently. Consider how your values and worldview underpin all communication. Think of how you manage situations where you are challenged to emotionally regulate before and during engagement with people. What support do you need from others and what permissions do you need to give yourself to make it more possible for you to experience positive outcomes?

You can reproduce this table for your own reflection.

| Micro-skills | What example do I have of these skills in action? | What aspects of these skills do I need to improve? | Where and with whom will I try to improve these skills? | How will I know when I have improved these skills? |
|---|---|---|---|---|
| Planning ahead for communication | | | | |
| Self-regulation – verbal and non-verbal | | | | |
| Taking the 'adult' role | | | | |
| Nodding in a timely way | | | | |
| Appropriate use of posture | | | | |
| Changing my approach due to a person's age, stage, cognitive ability | | | | |

→

| Micro-skills | What example do I have of these skills in action? | What aspects of these skills do I need to improve? | Where and with whom will I try to improve these skills? | How will I know when I have improved these skills? |
|---|---|---|---|---|
| 'Reading the tone' and responding to mirror it | | | | |
| 'Reading the tone' and actively responding to change this | | | | |
| Eye contact that says that I am listening | | | | |
| Eye contact that says I agree | | | | |
| Eye contact that shows empathy | | | | |
| Eye contact that does not show I am triggered (= good self-regulation) | | | | |
| Eye contact that expresses disagreement | | | | |
| Paraphrasing | | | | |
| Reframing the person's statements helpfully | | | | |
| Summarising the information given by the person | | | | |
| Neutral facial expressions | | | | |

| Micro-skills | What example do I have of these skills in action? | What aspects of these skills do I need to improve? | Where and with whom will I try to improve these skills? | How will I know when I have improved these skills? |
|---|---|---|---|---|
| Minimal use of 'fillers' in communication, eg 'er', 'em', 'you know', 'like' | | | | |
| Negotiation | | | | |
| Meeting people 'where they are at' | | | | |
| Communicating in a way that maintains awareness of personal emotional boundaries | | | | |
| Repeating chunks of information to ensure the other person understands | | | | |
| Checking the person understands | | | | |
| Holding back from giving advice when empathy and validation are needed instead | | | | |
| Validating the person, their feelings or their situation: 'It seems like…' 'It sounds like…' 'It looks like…' | | | | |

→

| Micro-skills | What example do I have of these skills in action? | What aspects of these skills do I need to improve? | Where and with whom will I try to improve these skills? | How will I know when I have improved these skills? |
|---|---|---|---|---|
| Breathing or pausing (giving space to think) before speaking | | | | |
| Using open questions | | | | |
| Using reflective questions | | | | |
| Affirming attributes, strengths and efforts | | | | |
| Disagreeing with someone in a way that does not shame them | | | | |
| Saying 'no' without saying the word 'no' | | | | |
| Challenging someone respectfully | | | | |
| Using language that shows I value and appre-ciate others' knowledge and practice | | | | |
| Articulating options clearly | | | | |
| Keeping quiet when I want to speak | | | | |

| Micro-skills | What example do I have of these skills in action? | What aspects of these skills do I need to improve? | Where and with whom will I try to improve these skills? | How will I know when I have improved these skills? |
|---|---|---|---|---|
| Speaking when I want to keep quiet | | | | |
| Matching the tempo of emotion without matching the negativity of emotion, then slowing pace of speech to help the other person regulate | | | | |
| Holding my thoughts and waiting for the other person to stop speaking before I start speaking | | | | |
| Leading conversations appropriately | | | | |
| Knowing when to interrupt someone | | | | |
| Knowing when to end the conversation | | | | |

*Target skills improvement continuously*. Scrutinise what you perceive you are doing right as well as what you perceive you are doing 'wrong'. Study other people's communication to see what they do well and copy what works into your own toolbox of techniques.

*Name it, tame it and claim it*. Bring micro-skills into your awareness. Value small changes and adopt improvements into your established practice style.

# CASE STUDY 1: MARK

## Background

Mark is a very handsome 15-year-old boy who can sing beautifully and play the flute by ear. He makes friends easily and can entertain a room full of people, commanding attention with his good nature and charisma. Mark's mother died of a brain tumour when Mark was 13. Extended family became involved and he went to live with his, thus far, estranged father. Mark's dad had been a street busker all his adult life, sometimes sleeping rough, sometimes 'sofa-surfing'. When Mark went to live with him, his father had settled into a house they could call their own. However, Mark's father did not prioritise education and quickly saw that Mark's singing talent could bring extra cash working with him on the street. Mark's behaviour at school also led to him being placed in off-site education provision. In effect, Mark had only been to school at the start of each term in the preceding year, preferring to spend his time singing on the street for money.

Mark's dad treated Mark as an equal adult rather than a child. This meant that he did not protect his son in the way that Mark needed him to. Mark was exposed to the lifestyle his father had prior to Mark coming into his care. A lot of adults who lived a transient lifestyle would come and stay at the house, sometimes having parties. Cannabis was often smoked and soon Mark also began smoking cannabis. Mark would be sent for errands by friends of his dad in return for pocket money. Along the way, one of his dad's friends had also persuaded Mark to have sex with him for money. It is unclear whether Mark's dad knew about this at the time, but Mark saw this as a way of making his own money to buy cannabis and other drugs. Education professionals were very concerned about Mark missing school, which led to investigation of the family circumstances and Mark coming to live in residential care.

## Today's events

We had all been at the beach: three staff and three young people (Mark and two girls, Shauna and Mikaela). It was a lovely sunny day, and it was really good to see the young people being children. They were paddling in and out of the waves and throwing a ball to each other. Mark had drawn some children on the beach, younger than himself, into the games and they all had fun.

Mark had worn long shorts with nothing on his top half (and had brought a change of clothes). Mark was proud of his body and needed to be advised on not drawing attention to himself among the families on the beach. He was excited and using a lot of energy to run around. He was quick witted and loudly vocal in the group. He needed to be taken aside and advised that his sexualised comment to the fathers of one of the younger children was not okay. He did calm down a bit but still made sexualised gestures when we were having juice and crisps on the blankets. This would have been noticeable to members of the public and Mark had been warned that if he continued we would head home.

Shauna needed the toilet, so June (a care worker) went with her. The changing huts were a bit of a distance from the water. Shortly, Mikaela said she needed the toilet too and as she also needed an escort Frances went with her. This meant that I was left with Mark on the beach by myself. They had all been gone a long time, and I tried to call June by phone to check if everything was alright. No answer.

I made my way to the top of the sand dunes where I could see the toilet block. I could see Mark at the same time, or so I thought – I looked round and he wasn't there! I ran back down to the main beach to ask other people where he had gone. A couple of minutes later, Mark appeared from the nearby dunes, looking wide-eyed and agitated but trying to be nonchalant. At the same time, June called back on the phone, saying that they had lost Shauna.

## Questions

- What should I say to Mark as something was clearly not right?

- How should I support June, who was really worried that Shauna had disappeared?

- How do we find Shauna?

- How do we ensure that Mikaela's needs are considered and that the impact of events is lessened for her?

- How can we get everyone home safely as we have only got one car – and I don't have the keys?

## My practice

| | My practice | Why did I do this? |
|---|---|---|
| 1 | I clarified on the phone that June had called the police and to be honest I cut the conversation a bit short with her, explaining that I needed to talk with Mark. | I could see that Mark was highly anxious – this was out of the norm for him, and he needed my attention. |
| 2 | I asked Mark gently if he was okay. I felt myself becoming anxious as I had been supposed to be looking after him and I had taken my eyes off him. | I didn't want to come across as angry with him even though I thought that his behaviour was going to make it appear as though I had not looked after him properly.<br><br>I thought that he needed a kind and neutral approach, so I worked hard at this. |

| | My practice | Why did I do this? |
|---|---|---|
| 3 | I said to Mark, *'Where did you go? – I looked round and couldn't see you!'* He responded that he had *'just been for a slash'* (I took this to mean that he had urinated in the sand dunes). I said that he could have easily gone to the toilets – we could have walked across. I said that it was not okay for people to go to the toilet outdoors. It is not hygienic and not safe. | I knew it is against the law in this country to urinate in a public place but as Mark was agitated, we could come back to this discussion later.<br><br>I did sense that a bit of my own anxiety was coming through so needed to take control of my thoughts and tone. |
| 4 | I said we should pack up the bag and get to the car. I said that June had phoned to say she was heading there too (which was partially true). | I needed to ensure Mark's safety. I was alarmed with his presentation but needed to help him regulate. The activity of packing up gave us a focus in the moment (albeit Mark appeared a bit dissociated). |
| 5 | I asked Mark if he wanted to sit down but he was quite lively – there was no way he was sitting here. | I did not know what had happened in the sand dunes but was clear that Mark's presentation was vastly different now from when he went into the dunes. |
| 6 | I asked him again if he was okay or if something had happened. He said, *'I only went for a slash.'* | I needed to figure out how concerned I should be to help me decide what to do next. |
| 7 | We walked towards the car together and Mark remained agitated. Sometimes his eyes darted around involuntarily. I asked him if he was looking for someone. He denied this. I decided to stop questioning him and work on calming him down. | There would need to be further questions asked but I should concentrate on restoring his sense of safety by being a dependable adult. |

→

| | My practice | Why did I do this? |
|---|---|---|
| 8 | We found both of the other care workers at the car and Mikaela was with them. June explained to Mark that Shauna had disappeared, and the police were on their way. This made Mark very anxious, and we immediately made a plan along with the young people that June would stay at the beachfront so if Shauna reappeared, she would be there for her, and the rest of us would all go home. | This seemed the most practical thing to do to calm the situation down and meet all of the children's needs.<br><br>This left June without a car, but we could sort that out. |
| 9 | Mikaela could see that Mark was agitated and said to him, *'What's with you?!'* | This could have wound Mark up further. |
| 10 | I put Mikaela in the front seat and Frances assumed she would be the driver as she had the keys. I seated myself diagonally opposite Frances. | This was so that I could give attention to Mark for continuity of care and also make it less likely for Mark to be able to grab Mikaela if she made a comment he did not like. |
| 11 | Through non-verbal communication between myself and Frances, she realised that all was not well with Mark and me, albeit she did not ask verbally. I led the conversation in the car on the journey. | I led so that I could help keep away from topics of conversation that Mikaela did not need to be involved in, and to help co-regulate with Mark as he was still very tense. We needed to get home without any further issues. |
| 12 | I suggested we get comfortable after tea and spend the rest of the evening watching a film as we had had such a busy day and it had been so sunny. We discussed film options until we arrived back safely. | Planning ahead, I knew that workers' time would be needed to help with Shauna (hopefully she will be found safely). Yet we still had to speak with Mark by himself about what had happened in the few minutes he was out of my sight. It would be difficult to facilitate more activities with the group with such a lot needing to be done. On the journey, talking about mundane things seemed to be a distraction. |

# How might these theories apply to the situation?

• Need

• Mentalisation

• Trauma

# How might these models of intervention apply?

• Crisis intervention

• Co-regulation

• Secure base

# Reflective questions for me as a worker

1. Could I have done anything differently?

2. Can I forgive myself for taking my eyes off Mark?

3. What advice would I give another worker in this situation, and can I take some of that advice on board myself?

4. How will I approach the conversation I must have with Mark now we are safely back home?

5. Who else can help now?

# Reflective questions for the team

1. What risks were present when we decided to take these three young people out together and did we risk assess correctly?

2. Did we know these young people well enough to inform our decision to take them on this outing?

3. Is there anything else that we could have prepared in advance to prevent this situation from occurring?

4. Should we have decided to come home earlier when Mark was making loud sexualised comments?

5. What other learning comes out of this?

6. How can we support each other as a team?

# CASE STUDY 2: ZANITA

## Background

Zanita is a very intelligent 14-year-old girl with a sharp sense of humour. She is a talented horse rider and avid reader who enjoys classic books and period dramas. She also finds it difficult to trust people. When Zanita was a toddler, her mother had prioritised her own desires to continue in relationships with male partners over her responsibility as a parent and had handed Zanita over to the care of her grand-mother while she left the country. She returned after a couple of years, set up home with a different partner and began to spend time with Zanita's grandmother. They often bought and sold second-hand goods together and went to yard sales and thrift shops with Zanita's older female cousins. Zanita's grandmother did not appear to be able to parent Zanita effectively as well as spend time with her daughter, so social services had become involved with the family. Zanita had been placed with four successive foster families before her placement in residential care. Zanita was anxious around the limited online contact she had with her family, who lived around a hundred miles away from the placement. She wanted her clothes ironed and her hair to be shiny and pristine before every online session. The sessions were supervised to offer Zanita emotional reassurance, as relationships were strained and she had never been observed sharing any of her many achievements with her family.

## Today's events

My care worker colleague Jack was agitated. He was pacing around the house looking for his ring. He had been openly showing it to the young people earlier and letting them handle it and try it on. He had been given it by his grandmother who had recently passed away and he realised he did not now have it in his possession.

Zanita had a sparkle in her eyes. She had a reasonable relationship with Jack and knew him well. He challenged her that she knew where his ring was. She made a play of checking under cushions and down the side of the furniture. Jack and another colleague, Martin, continued to search. Jack was becoming more agitated, again asking Zanita to tell him where the ring was. She denied know-ledge. Then without warning, she suddenly started to become anxious and angry, rapidly escalating to throwing things around. She was seething with aggression, calling Jack all the bad things she could think of, marching around, pulling the curtains down and upending the furniture. I silently called for some assistance from other workers.

Martin (care worker) tried to engage verbally with Zanita to attempt to de-escalate her behaviours and keep her away from the other four young people who were around and who could see and feel the tension mounting. Martin asked Zanita to take some time in her room to relax and, with some initial refusal and further cajoling, she moved closer to her room but not into it. She was screaming and swearing at Jack. Sue, my other care worker colleague, tried to help regulate the emotions of the other young people by distracting and moving them away, as they too were starting to become agitated.

## Questions

- How should I support Jack, who was very tense, and then being verbally targeted by Zanita?

- What could I contribute (in the role I hold) to helping my other peers?

- Do I need to support the other young people present so that the situation does not escalate further with them?

- How can I use my relationships or relational skills to de-escalate this situation?

## My practice

| | My practice | Why did I do this? |
|---|---|---|
| 1 | I carefully observed the other children. They appeared relatively manageable for Sue, and Jack had gone over to join them. I said gently to him, *'The ring can't have gone anywhere out of the building. We will find it.'* I then shut the door to the living area and went to Zanita. | I had wanted to provide some privacy for Zanita to compose herself as well as put some physical distance between her and the rest of the young people in case any of them became the target of her frustrations. I did not want Zanita to see Jack as his presence was likely to trigger her again. Also, I was unclear whether he saw that he had just created an avoidable situation by not safeguarding his ring as per policy on staff belongings, and I didn't know if he was going to continue pressing Zanita again to disclose where it was. If so, I didn't want to leave the chance for further escalation. |
| 2 | I stood calmly and observed. | In the seconds I was engaged with Jack, other workers were speaking with Zanita, and I needed to figure out the position before being able to add anything helpful. |
| 3 | Gary, the worker leading the interaction with Zanita, was pursuing compliance, saying that if Zanita did not go to her room things would become worse for her. Zanita was scowling, very tense and refusing to move. Although she was sitting on the floor, I kept a standing distance from her, like the other two workers present. | Zanita's verbal pitch was increasing, and I thought she might lash out. |

| | My practice | Why did I do this? |
|---|---|---|
| 4 | I nodded to Gary and quietly tried to interject. He didn't stop me.<br><br>(Zanita stopped screaming and sat there seething with anger and adrenaline.) | This subtle body language was a recognised signal between workers that there was an agreed change of tack. I really didn't know what this was until I started speaking but I could see that Gary was not getting very far with gaining compliance. Maybe we jointly recognised that he had moved into 'cause and effect' discussions rather than using 'regulate and relate' as first-intervention steps before 'reasoning' (see Perry, 2011 on p. 106). Whether Gary recognised this or not, we both understood that we could work together to support the direction of discussion. |
| 5 | I said in what I hoped was a neutral tone, *'I am not sure what happened in there, just now, but it seems like big feelings have been triggered for you. We don't want to put you under pressure – it's not necessary just now for you to explain. The only thing I can figure out is that there will be logical reasons for why things went the way they did just now. And... one thing is for sure, if any one of us* [I nodded to indicate Gary and James (care workers)] *had the experiences you have had, then we may have reacted in the same way to whatever the trigger was.'* | I did not know if the other workers knew about Zanita having been abandoned by first her mother, then her grandmother, then her four disrupted foster placements. I had hypothesised in my head that she may have been triggered as Jack was clearly fond of his grandmother and Zanita might have longed for a relationship where anyone (grandmother or not) meant so much to her with the level of care and attachment that Jack had shown. Perhaps this might have been a reminder of what she did not have.<br><br>However, I did not know this for sure and did not need the detail confirmed for me to respond in a way that could neutralise the situation and validate her as a person before trying to help her regulate further.<br><br>I believed that if Gary had carried on pressing Zanita to go to her room, she would have experienced further abandonment and rejection and may have assaulted the other young people or us, which would have required physical intervention.<br><br>I figured that she needed workers to co-regulate with her. |
| 6 | My reframing of the situation seemed to take Zanita off guard, especially as the other workers were agreeing. I still stood back. | She did not need anyone physically close as this may have been overwhelming for her. She must still have had adrenaline in her body and had not yet returned to her baseline functioning. I didn't want to trigger her by coming closer. |

$\longrightarrow$

| | My practice | Why did I do this? |
|---|---|---|
| 7 | I said, '*It's probably a lot easier to put the furniture back and fix the curtains than it is to feel the big feelings.*'<br><br>I turned to Gary and James and asked, '*Would you agree?*' (They saw that this was slightly helping as Zanita was becoming stiller and not shouting any more. They nodded and agreed.) | This was to validate Zanita's emotions, make her feel heard and supported but without trying to name the pre-cipitating issue or triggering her to feel further shame.<br><br>I drew in the other adults to the conversation so that Zanita could feel that everyone was 'on her side' and we could support her together to de-escalate the situation. I thought that there would be plenty of time when she was calm to talk through what she could have done dif-ferently and provide space for her to understand her own triggers and 'window of tolerance'. |
| 8 | I said, '*We need to help you move on from this. To be honest there have been plenty of times when I have done things I later regret – and I can't speak for "these two"* [I smiled and nodded a little towards Gary and James] *but I am guessing they have done stuff in the spur of the moment that wasn't really the best deci-sion. But people come through it and carry on.*' Gary nodded and James left the area as he saw that he was not needed to help de-escalating. | This was to take things one step further to provide Zanita with confirming evidence that all the adults present were nurturing, rather than leaving her with any thoughts that they might be condemning or rejecting her as a person (as she may well have experienced from adults in the past).<br><br>My half smile was to help Zanita relax a little. I was careful of the timing of this so that she experienced it as supportive and friendly. A few minutes ago, when she was more agitated, that might have triggered her to act aggressively.<br><br>If someone was hurt in the previous incident or the impact on others had been greater, I would have needed to take different decisions though. |
| 9 | I saw that Zanita was responding by calming down so I said, '*Can we park this all for now and take a breather? We have got lots of time. Have you got a pen? I want to draw you something.*' | I didn't think we really did have lots of time as the other young people needed me to facilitate activities for them. However, it would be worse if Zanita re-joined the group still adrenalised as things might escalate a second time. I did not know if the other children might target Zanita if they thought she had hidden the sentimental ring from Jack.<br><br>I wanted to get Zanita in her room, provide a distrac-tion and give her some time to return to her baseline regulation.<br><br>I also needed to reassure her that she was important enough to receive adults' time as she had experienced so much rejection in the past. |

| | My practice | Why did I do this? |
|---|---|---|
| 10 | She nodded to the table in her room we could both see, although she didn't move. I asked, 'Can I get it?' She shrugged – which I took as agreement. I got it and a piece of paper. I said, 'Can we sit in here for a bit with the door open?' I began to draw a mandala. | I was looking for her agreement in a way that gave her power.<br><br>From this point I was reasonably sure that the situation could be resolved. We could discuss the ring a bit later and hold her accountable if and when the facts were established. We could also return to the learning points around managing triggers when Zanita had time to process things and was ready to reflect.<br><br>I was sure that we did not need to pick over the detail of why she had reacted in this way, unless she was ready to discuss this. We could test the water on this later. I just planned to help her devise her own strategies that would be more effective when the 'big feelings' came. |

## How might these theories apply to the situation?

• Unconditional positive regard

• Attachment

• Identity

• Loss and change

• Need

• Resilience

## How might these models of intervention apply?

• Secure base

• Opportunity-led practice

• Strengths-based practice

## Reflective questions for me as a worker

1. What about this situation did I find triggering?

2. How do I manage to regulate my own feelings and behaviour when I am triggered?

3. How would I have worked with the other adults present if they did not appear to be allowing me to lead in the direction I did?

4. In what other situations could I use the technique of validating a young person's feelings when I could only guess at the reasons for their behaviour?

5. What will I prepare to say to Zanita when she is calm enough to have a reflective discussion about her reactions and behaviour?

## Reflective questions for the team

1. How has early years neglect impacted Zanita's current functioning?

2. How could we ensure that everyone working with Zanita is aware of what might trigger her and how best to respond?

3. When Zanita began throwing things around, did we act calmly and decisively as a team to de-escalate the situation? (What helped and what hindered?)

4. Was our decision making clear to the young people watching the situation unfold with Zanita and did we help them feel as safe as possible?

5. How can we support and nurture Jack as a team, rather than shame him during the debriefing discussion (which will need to acknowledge his mistake of not following policy and leaving his ring in a safe place)?

# CASE STUDY 3: MILLIE

## Background

Millie is a 13-year-old girl who likes to watch soap operas and romantic comedies on Netflix. She is the youngest of a family of six sisters. Millie has spent time living in the family home with a different combination of sisters at any one time throughout her life. Millie's aunt also lived with them for two years with her daughter. During this time, one of Millie's sisters was rehabilitated home from foster care as her aunt was considered a protective factor to support Millie's mother who had periodic mental health difficulties. There were no males ever known to have lived with the family and Millie's mother has repeatedly and openly said that she sought pregnancy rather than relationships with males. About a year ago, there was a fire in the house where Millie, two sisters and their mother needed to evacuate in the middle of the night. Although no one was hurt, this was a very frightening experience for them all. The family lost a lot of their belongings and had to spend some time in temporary accommodation before they were rehoused. The sister closest to Millie in age was suspected of starting this fire deliberately and is currently in living in a separate residential care facility in a neighbouring county.

Millie has lived in residential care with us for about five months. She behaves impeccably when she spends time with adults but does not like people her own age. She is considerably behind her peers in terms of academic learning and is likely to have an IQ which is lower than average. Millie lacks motivation and has poor self-care skills. She often needs to be prompted to shower and change her clothes. If not checked, she will wear the same clothes day after day. This needs careful monitoring to ensure that Millie is not targeted by other young people for her poor presentation.

## Today's events

Millie's oldest sister was supposed to come to visit her today. However, her boyfriend's car had broken down on the motorway and they had to be towed to the garage. Millie found this out after the time of her scheduled visit and had been left waiting all afternoon wondering why her sister had not appeared. Workers had tried to call her sister a few times, but she was not answering her phone. Millie was silent when she was told that her sister would not make it to visit her today.

Millie had eaten her tea without talking much. I had tried to engage Millie in making plans for playing board games in the evening, but she was not interested. This was not unusual though. There had then been a heated argument between two other young people in the house. While this was being de-escalated by workers, Millie poured all the milk from the fridge into the kitchen sink and sunk her hands into it. There was quite a lot of milk, so the level reached well above the cuffs of her jumper. Millie stood there moving her hands around like they were swimming. She began finger painting in milk around the wall above the sink with milk dripping off her clothes.

Alex (a young person) noticed this and began sneering at Millie: *'What are you doing you weirdo?! – who even does that? You would think that you are two years old – ma – ma – want a dummy?'* Nick (another young person) came bounding into the kitchen and started shouting: *'What have you done that for? She's wasted all the milk – I wanted that – other people wanted that. You're thick as mince, ya total spanner!'*

# Questions

- How can I meet Millie's and Nick's differing needs for nurture at the same time?

- How can I address Alex and Nick, who are targeting Millie with insults?

- Knowing that Millie does not care about how clean she is, how do I help her regulate her emotions and stop this behaviour?

- How do I encourage her to change into clean dry clothes?

- How do I steer the group to more productive use of their time?

# My practice

| | My practice | Why did I do this? |
|---|---|---|
| 1 | Amanda (care worker) came into the kitchen, and I said to Nick that I would get more milk from the big fridge, as there was plenty in there. | Nick needed to be reassured, given his own background of poverty and deprivation, that the supplies would not run out.<br><br>Even if Amanda was intending saying this to him as well, I thought it would do no harm for him to hear this consistently. |
| 2 | In a split second it needed to be decided which worker would talk with which young person. I was nearest Millie so, without turning my back on Alex, I saw that Amanda was engaging with him. I made eye contact with Daniel (care worker) and indicated that he should also assist. | I knew that Simon (care worker) was still dealing with one of the other young people who had exchanged heated words with Alex a minute ago and Daniel was on the phone. Without knowing Alex and Nick too well, I thought it would have helped for each young person to have an adult engaging with them individually at that time. |
| 3 | Amanda reassured Nick too that more milk was available and managed to encourage him out of the kitchen. Millie continued to finger paint. I pulled the plug out of the sink and let the milk drain away. Millie did not speak or react. | I pulled the plug out of the sink to reduce the options for Millie's current behaviour and to be the adult in the room. – I realised this could have gone either way – de-escalate or escalate. She silently continued to make marks on the wall with the milk that had soaked into her jumper. |

| | My practice | Why did I do this? |
|---|---|---|
| 4 | Daniel was struggling to engage Alex effectively and he was continuing to make 'baby' noises towards Millie. I ignored Alex and focused my attention on Millie. | Although Daniel was struggling with Alex, I had confidence that he would manage, as he has a good relationship with Alex.<br><br>I considered that Millie was communicating a need for attention. If I had given my attention to Alex, it may have increased both his and Millie's behaviours. |
| 5 | Millie did well to ignore Alex too and she pretended to be fixated on her milk drawings. I got some kitchen roll and tore off bits to drop on the floor to mop up the milk. I said, *'Here, let me help you.'* I gently patted the kitchen roll on Millie's elbow to catch the drips. She carried on squeezing a bit more milk out of her jumper. | I tried to dry the milk on the floor first to stop us both slipping. Safety first! I also thought that Millie was needing to feel cared for and that she was asking for it in this way. She accepted my gentle gesture of drying her elbow. I didn't clean her milk drawings immediately as I thought this might invalidate her emotional state when she wanted this to be recognised. |
| 6 | Alex left the kitchen of his own accord, possibly as he was not getting his desired reaction from Millie. When he and Daniel left, she started a new movement of flicking milk. I said, *'I am staying with you, Millie.'* | I thought this was a kind of test from Millie about what I would tolerate. I thought that there was only milk on the walls and surfaces, and nobody was getting physically hurt. I was mindful that she may have felt abandoned by her sister. |
| 7 | I said, *'It looks like some confusing things have happened today. Am I guessing right?'*<br><br>I dropped my eye gaze to the cupboards and leaned back slightly. | I wanted to validate what Millie might be feeling, at the same time as offering some words around emotions that might fit – not to put words into her mouth but to make a suggestion to test it out. I thought if the emotion could be named its power could be reduced.<br><br>I moved and looked away so that she might perceive me as non-threatening while she processed this. |
| 8 | She said, *'No, I am angry and sad.'* I asked, *'About Katie?'* and she nodded. She flicked milk with a bit more vigour. *'She never phoned me – she left me hanging.'*<br><br>I said, *'Anyone in your position might have felt disappointed.'* I waited. | I thought it might help if her feelings were normalised and to give her time to think this through. Acknowledging her position may have supported her self-regulation. |

| | My practice | Why did I do this? |
|---|---|---|
| 9 | She said, '*I always phone her and if I was meant to visit her, I would let her know what was happening. She is a fat cow.*' I didn't check her for her language. I said, '*I have seen you phoning her, yes.*' I just waited. | As Millie was not really doing any harm, I thought it would be more productive continuing the conversation here while she was sort of engaged with something. The other workers had successfully taken the other young people through to the other room so there was no pressing need to move her on.<br><br>I validated what she said and just gave her space to think or to talk. |
| 10 | I offered her a piece of kitchen roll without suggesting what she might do with it. She screwed it up and threw it on the floor and jumped up and down on it. She grabbed another and did the same. And another, and another. | I considered doing the same as her and turning it into fun but thought that this might escalate things. Too soon! She needed an adult response. |
| 11 | I started cleaning up the surfaces and she said, '*I hate her.*' I said, '*I can see that she has let you down.*'<br><br>She was starting to calm down now that she was speaking openly. I asked, '*I know we can't turn back the clock, but what can we do for you just now to help you feel a bit better?*' '*Nothing!*' she said, '*I want to phone my mum!*'<br><br>I stopped cleaning up and said, '*Okay, let's pop your jumper in the wash and call your mum.*' | When she had asked to call her mum, I prioritised this. The cleaning could happen a little bit later. I thought that it was important for her to believe she had been heard and that I was going to act on her wishes promptly. I realised that the attachment she had with her family members was driving her behaviours and I wanted to help meet her emotional needs. I also wanted to help keep the evening running smoothly for the whole group. However, reflecting ahead, I really did want her to change out of the wet jumper now as, if the call to her mum did not go as she wanted it to, she may have refused to hand it over. |

## How might these theories apply to the situation?

• Attachment

• Systems

• Loss and change

• Emotional intelligence

• Transactional analysis

## How might these models of intervention apply?

• Secure base

• Co-regulation

• Trauma-sensitive practice

## Reflective questions for me as a worker

1. How might things have gone differently if I had gone and wiped the milk off the walls immediately?

2. Would there have been another way to respond to this with a different young person?

3. If Alex refused to leave the kitchen, would I have needed to do anything else to care for Millie?

4. What support do I need and from whom now that the immediate issue has been resolved?

## Reflective questions for the team

1. How might the gender of the worker leading with Millie have affected the outcome?

2. How have family systems potentially impacted Millie's current functioning?

3. Did we work as a team to de-escalate the situation? (What helped and what hindered?)

4. How could I have framed options in a more appealing way to Millie if she refused to hand over her wet jumper for washing?

# CASE STUDY 4: STEWART

## Background

Stewart is a 17-year-old boy who likes motorbikes. He can draw parts and name them all. He can accurately describe how to remove a central drive cam chain and a carburetor. He studies motorbike manuals in his room and has covered his walls with posters of different bikes. Stewart has an aptitude for maths and physics but had believed that he was 'too cool for school' and did not study for exams.

He began to come to the attention of police when he was around age 15. His dad and uncle had two lock-up garages next to each other and were running a small enterprise fixing motorbikes and cars and selling them on. There were complaints from nearby residential neighbours of anti-social behaviour, where like-minded friends were gathering at the lock-ups and blaring loud music. Stewart and some other friends his age had been found there drinking alcohol with the adults.

Social work became more involved with the family after Stewart's mum crashed her car, resulting in a brain injury and reduced movement in her left arm. Stewart's two younger sisters were then cared for away from home (they did not have the same father) and Stewart stayed with his mum. To cope with pain, Stewart's mum began using illicit substances, and Stewart took on a caring role for her. Stewart's dad became aware of his ex-partner's use of substances and began giving Stewart maintenance money directly. Stewart found himself with more money than he could imagine and began dealing in motorbike spares like his dad. He was clever and made some money. At age 16, he was apprehended by police several times due to riding motorbikes in inappropriate places. It was also thought that he was vulnerable due to his association with people who were suspected of money laundering.

Stewart came to residential care with us a year ago and had a very poor attitude towards authority. He did not like the police as they had seized his motorbike and he did not like being told what to do. Roughly every third word Stewart said was a swear word (these have been omitted in the outline of the exchange below!). Stewart cared deeply about his mum and became anxious when he did not know what was going on at home.

## Today's events

Stewart had been home to see his mum and returned to our care as previously agreed. He was chatty as normal and, predictably, he was not pleased with the attitude of the conductor on the train. We had a chat about the man just doing his job and that other people would get their clothes dirty if he had put his shoes on the seats. Nothing out of the ordinary. This arrangement of Stewart travelling back and forth had been mainly working well for a couple of months every second weekend, and the longer-term plan was for him to get a flat close to his mum's house. However, shortly after he came back today, he pressed a button on his phone by mistake in front of me and another young person and it played a message from his mum alluding to the fact that he had previously given her money and she expected him to bring some again when he saw her.

# Questions

- Is it my business as a care worker what money Stewart has, where it has come from and what he does with it?

- Is Stewart's mum exploiting him?

- What don't I know, and what do I need to know?

- What are the risks and protective factors?

- Given that Stewart likes to be autonomous, how will I handle this?

- How will I handle the needs of the other young person who now knows this information?

## My practice

| | My practice | Why did I do this? |
|---|---|---|
| 1 | When we clearly heard the message Stewart's mum had left, the other young person sniggered and said, '*Your mum is strapped for cash, Stewart – sort it out!*' Stewart made it clear that he did not appreciate his peer's comments. I shook my head and said, '*That sounds like a private message that Stewart didn't mean us to hear. Can we check the list to see whose turn it is to help us cook tonight? I am thinking that we might be out of cheese so we need to pop and get some, or decide what else we can have.*' | I was buying a little bit of time to think what to do. As the other young person was there, I did not think it right to question Stewart any further at that minute. I also did not want an argument escalating between the boys. |
| 2 | We carried on with the evening and in a quiet moment I let my co-worker know what had happened. Together we decided that I would speak with Stewart. | I let my co-worker know in case the situation was referred to by either of the boys during the evening. I thought it best that she was also prepared to understand how to respond to anything emerging over the course of the evening. |

| | My practice | Why did I do this? |
|---|---|---|
| | | As the message was played in front of me, we both agreed that it would be best for me to follow it up. If my co-worker knew I was doing this, she could also distract other young people, but be ready to help me should I need support. |
| 3 | Later when I was in the living room alone with Stewart, I asked him gently, *'What was that about earlier when you played the message from your mum? Is everything okay?'* | I needed to start finding out what risks were around for Stewart so we could figure the best way to care for him. |
| 4 | He replied, *'Nothing, its fine. It's fine.'*<br><br>I paused so as to seem non-confrontational. | I wanted him to feel supported rather than under scrutiny as I was aware of his preference for self-sufficiency. |
| 5 | I said, *'I am wondering about your mum's health. How was she keeping this weekend?'* | I wanted to show empathy towards his mum, whom I know he is very attached to and worries about. |
| 6 | He said, *'She's fine – she just sometimes needs a little bit extra. She will be fine if I can get a flat soon.'*<br><br>I made a comment about something on the TV then said, *'I am not sure what you mean by needing a little bit extra.'* At the same time I pushed the bowl of crisps towards him, as if offering him some if he wanted. | I wanted to keep the conversation open until I could be clear about what the issues were.<br><br>I tried to soften the conversation with a reference to the TV rather than seem to be interrogating him with one question after the other.<br><br>I knew he could already reach the crisps if he wanted, but I tried to offer a gesture of openness and friendliness so he could perceive me as non-threatening. |
| 7 | He said, *'She is sore all the time. She needs fixing up.'*<br><br>I said, *'So are you meaning she needs to buy more medication?'* | I took this to mean that Stewart's mum had asked him for money to fund her illicit substance use. I did not want to say this outright as it may have shut the conversation down. I was alert to the dilemma Stewart was in and how powerless he may have felt. This would not have sat well with him, as he saw himself as having a high level of self-efficacy. |

$\longrightarrow$

| | My practice | Why did I do this? |
|---|---|---|
| 8 | I said, *'Is she needing to see the doctor again so they can review her pain medication?'*<br><br>He stared hard at the TV and became tense.<br><br>He said, *'Doctors do nothing. I will fix it. Can you email my social worker about my flat? Find out what's happening?'*<br><br>I said, *'I can email her, yes, and I can see you are worried about your mum. And I am worried about you. Listen, does your dad know that your mum is in this much pain?'* | I wanted to offer a practical solution that Stewart could think about. We both knew that we could not make Stewart's mum go to the doctor. I appreciated that Stewart liked 'fixing' things and that his approach was likely to be linked to his learning style as well as his dislike of authority and his attachment to his mum.<br><br>As he was not shutting down the conversation, I thought it best to probe a little bit more to find out any other risks to Stewart. |
| 9 | He said, *'He knows nothing. You can't tell him.'* He looked genuinely horrified. I reassured him. *'It's not my place to say anything about this to your dad, Stewart. I am just concerned for you and the position you are in. I do think we should tell your social worker you are worried though. She might be able to go and check on your mum.'*<br><br>He relaxed a bit and said, *'Whatever. She will be fine.'* | I kept the direction of conversation around tackling the root cause (Stewart's worry about his mum) rather than the symptom of the money and where this was coming from etc. I thought Stewart might become defensive and think that I was being punitive if I focused on his behaviours.<br><br>I thought that I had got agreement from him that his social worker should be informed but needed to make my intentions more explicit. |
| 10 | After a bit of a pause, and some more crisps each, I said, *'I will tell her you are worried, and I am worried. I will need to tell her that your mum needs extra money and sometimes you have been giving her this.'*<br><br>He looked directly at me. *'She's my mum and nobody can stop me. Tell her to get me a flat!'* | I stopped the conversation there as I needed to work out how to take this forward. I still did not know how much money he had been passing to his mum, nor much about her wider situation. I didn't know where the money was coming from although I suspected Stewart was getting it from his dad. I was satisfied for tonight that Stewart was talking about the issues he was facing and satisfied that others, including his social worker, could help mitigate risk. |

| | My practice | Why did I do this? |
|---|---|---|
| | I agreed to ask his social worker about a flat. | I saw future risks of Stewart being asked by his mum to go and get illicit substances for her, but that was not a conversation for today. |
| 11 | Much later on that evening, I spoke briefly with the other young person. This had also been planned between my co-worker and me. I reassured him that if he had any worries about anything he could come and talk but there would be no need for him to raise it with Stewart again. We talked about being respectful of others' privacy and that he could expect the same of his own business. | I thought I would keep an eye on his behaviour and see what the impact was on him and the relationship he had with Stewart.<br><br>I did not get into a conversation with him about me having spoken with Stewart, nor any action we would need to take as a staff team etc. |

## How might these theories apply to the situation?

• Attachment

• Rational choice

• Social constructionism

• Learning styles

• Loss and change

• Emotional intelligence

## How might these models of intervention apply?

• Opportunity-led practice

• Crisis intervention

⸱ De cooalation

• Task-centred practice

• Relationship-based practice

## Reflective questions for me as a worker:

1. What would have been different if I had spoken with both boys straight away?

2. What would have been different if my co-worker had spoken with Stewart?

3. What do we still not know about the risks?

4. Was there anything else I should have spoken with Stewart about?

5. Who else needs to be informed about the information gathered?

## Reflective questions for the team

1. It is our agency policy to sit and write case notes with the young person. What should we co-write about this situation?

2. What are the protective factors here?

3. What are the legal factors here?

4. What do we need to do to mitigate risk when Stewart goes home next time?

# CASE STUDY 5: PETER

## Background

Peter is 15 and enjoys football, both playing and watching. He dresses in the colours of his favourite football team. Ball skills take up a lot of his time and he even practises with a soft foam ball in his room. He is physically fit and likes going to the gym to use the rowing machines and the weights. He is competitive with himself, always trying to improve his personal best. He gets upset when he thinks he has not achieved what he set out to do and needs sensitive encouragement from workers. He idolises Matt, who is a personal trainer in his time outside work. He appreciates when others who are interested in fitness spend time with him and share their knowledge and tips.

Peter is biologically female and prior to coming into our care he was called Charlotte. He is openly transgender when speaking with staff but not yet trusting enough to share this with peers. He is going through the process of discovering his identity and is fiercely protective of his chosen pronouns. He is uncertain whether he is attracted to males or females or both. He is confused at times and has self-harmed by cutting his arms and the tops of his legs. He has not done this for a few weeks now, however, and is reflecting with the support of trusted staff (mainly just before bedtime) if he is attracted to Sienna, another young person in our care. He is unsure whether this is friendship or something more. He has made some tentative friendships with a couple of the other young people too and is wrestling with how to tell people (or if to tell people) that he is biologically female. Sienna has been accepting of Peter as he is and confided in him about her issues with her family. Although Peter is trying to process the concerning information she has shared, he considers her as a potential ally for himself.

We have been supporting Peter over the past six months in appointments with a consultant to get the information needed to prepare for hormone therapy. Peter chooses to bind his chest and has done for about a year. In his past he has been the victim of bullying due to his masculine presentation and his background.

Peter was previously assessed as a young carer, looking after his mum at age eight. He is the youngest of five siblings and there are 14 years between him and his next oldest sister. Three of his older brothers and sisters had left home by the time he was born, and he has never known his father. Peter's mum was 45 when she gave birth to Peter. She was subsequently diagnosed with a rare slow degenerative disease. Poverty and neglect were significant factors in his upbringing and Peter has developed some key survival thinking. His previous residential placement had passed on to us that they placed a snack box in Peter's room each night, as he had been found to be secreting and stockpiling extra food from the kitchen, albeit not eating it. We also adopted the food box idea and Peter seems to find it a comfort. We call it his 'power-pack', which he appears content with.

## Today's events

Peter's mum had visited him today. Peter had been nervous about this and after lengthy conversations it turned out that he did not want his peers to see his mum using her mobility scooter and walking frame. We went to some effort to facilitate this visit as Peter wished. Unfortunately, the time he and his mum spent together was very tense as she continued to call him Charlotte. She also gave him a piece of unsolicited information that his closest sister's father was actually someone the family had called an uncle. She thought Peter had known this, but he did not. It threw him into confusion. He was given emotional support after the visit but later that evening I found him with bleeding arms due to self-harm cuts. Sienna happened to be passing his door at that moment and was therefore aware of the situation.

## Questions

- What physical and psychological first aid should I give Peter?

- How can we utilise the trusting relationships Peter has with workers to help him manage his emotions safely?

- How can we ensure that the other children's needs, especially Sienna's, are met?

## My practice

| | My practice | Why did I do this? |
|---|---|---|
| 1 | I went into Peter's room. | I have a good relationship with him, and I had a duty of care and was motivated to see that he was safe and emotionally regulated. |
| 2 | I gently asked if he was okay and acknowledged that his cuts looked sore. | I wanted to reassure him and validate his pain. I wanted to use a humanistic approach to help him regulate. I have seen other workers be business-like and unsympathetic with young people who cut themselves and I strongly wanted to practise with unconditional positive regard. |
| 3 | Peter looked at the ground. I asked if he had cut himself any-where else. He shook his head. | I needed to assess what physical first aid he needed. |
| 4 | The cuts seemed like surface scratches, so I chatted for a minute to see what his mood was like and what risks were around for him. I told him what I was going to do and then went to get materials for cleaning up the cuts. | I assessed the risk before I left temporarily. This is the protocol for responding to this type of situation in our care setting. I was glad he knew I am reliable and that I would definitely return if I said I would, because we have a trusting relationship. |

| | My practice | Why did I do this? |
|---|---|---|
| 5 | On return, I asked if he wanted some help to clean his wounds. | If he did let me help, then I could get a closer look at his injuries. I also offered as it was a gesture of kindness and nurture. I left it open for him to decide if he wanted to accept the care from me. |
| 6 | He shook his head and took some sterile wipes. He then asked if Janine was working tonight in the other part of the care service. I said I could find out, but it would be best if he gave me the things that he had used to cut himself first before I checked. I said that I wanted him to be safe. | I needed to minimise the risk that he might cut himself again. I knew he liked Janine and I was happy to see if she was working. I was mindful that I would need to put parameters and boundaries in if she was able to come and speak with him, but I didn't want to say no straight away if there was a chance that he would hand over the sharps in anticipation of speaking with her. Any angle was worth a try to keep him safe, although this was a light touch and not a bargaining tool, of course. |
| 7 | Peter handed over some small shards of glass. I asked where he had got them from. He shrugged. I asked if there were more, and he dropped his eyes. I suspected it was likely that he had some more pieces. I did not push for him to give the glass to me. Instead, I said, *'From what I am seeing, I am thinking that you have been having a really difficult time.'* | If I demanded the extra pieces of glass, I thought we would end up in a polarised position. I wanted to acknowledge that I saw his intense emotions and validated them. This would be more likely to help de-escalate things. |
| 8 | Peter's eyes began to well up. He said, *'I don't know. I don't know anything. I would be better off not being born.'* I felt emotional as he did not deserve the situation that he was in. I gave a big pause and said, *'Well, I am glad you were born and that I am getting the chance to know you.'* | I paused so I could regulate my own emotions so I could then help him. I didn't really know what to say. I didn't want to say anything that made it worse, or pretend that I understood when I could not know the inner turmoil that he was facing. I knew that I would have the support of my seniors that it is okay not to know – to stay with the intensity but not have the answers. |

→

| | My practice | Why did I do this? |
|---|---|---|
| 9 | I gathered my thoughts and became a bit more confident in my not knowing stance, reflecting in the moment.<br><br>I said, '*I wish that it was all different for you. I wish I could make it different.*' | I wanted to be sensitive to the trauma and shock he was experiencing in real time about his identity relating to his mum's disclosure of who his sister's father was. I wanted to allude to a sense of validating the trauma that was in his background too. He and I had had many talks about his experiences. |
| 10 | As Bobby (care worker) was passing the open door, I said to him quietly, '*Listen, Peter just needs a minute or two.*' | I was mindful that the other care workers did not know what the situation was with Peter and might be wondering why I was so long in his room. This was unspoken code between us that things were 'okay but not okay', and I was asking Bobby to trust that I was doing what was needed to provide care to Peter. |
| 11 | I turned to Peter and said, '*I am going to have a cup of tea, would you like one?*' He shrugged.<br>I asked Bobby if he could bring us both tea if he got a moment, and '*perhaps a little slice of chocolate brownie?*' | I thought that I could show nurture by suggesting something to eat and drink as I knew this resonated with the way Peter liked to experience nurture. Even if he didn't want it just now, it was a gesture. |
| 12 | I stayed with Peter for a further 15 minutes or so. He asked, '*How do I know she is telling the truth?*' (He was referring to his mum's disclosure.) We chatted through what had been said when they spent time together. | I knew he needed some time with a safe adult, and I wanted to offer a secure base. I thought that if I did not give him time, he may cut himself again. |
| 13 | I asked him some open but sensitive questions and he was thoughtful, angry and upset in equal measure. | I was led by him and remained non-judgemental and what I thought was as trauma sensitive as I could be. I thought it was important to help him process some of his thoughts by offering to validate and contain his emotions. |
| 14 | Peter asked again if I could find out if Janine could come and see him. I called Janine from his room. There was no answer. I felt Peter's tension and that made me tense too. | I did not want to leave the room when he still had sharp items as I thought he might use them again. I thought it would help calm him if he could see that I was genuinely trying to contact Janine. |

| | My practice | Why did I do this? |
|---|---|---|
| 15 | I gently started kicking the foam ball against the wall. I continued chatting with Peter as he tried to make sense of things. | I was conscious that the length of time I was spending with Peter was perhaps leaving other young people with less care. I needed to try a different tactic to help Peter regulate so I could continue with other care tasks. |
| 16 | Eventually Peter chose to take over the ball and after another few minutes he handed me the glass. He seemed a bit more settled. | I did not want to second guess whether the ball skills gave Peter a sense of mastery and control to self-regulate, or if the ball was a distraction, or both. However, I was glad to have the sharps. |
| 17 | I said, 'Look, Sienna might be worried about you. I am thinking I should go and tell her that you are okay. What do you think?' | I had trusted that other care workers would reassure Sienna while I was with Peter, but it might also be comforting for Peter to perceive the possibility that Sienna would be concerned for him. It also gave him some choice in how his privacy was handled. |

## How might these theories apply to the situation?

• Assumptive world

• Stigma

• Loss and change

• Self-efficacy

• Identity

• Trauma

## How might these models of intervention apply?

• Life-story work (careful consideration of timing, planning and roles)

• Crisis intervention

• Mindfulness – or body-based work

• Social pedagogy

## Reflective questions for me as a worker

1. What would I have done if Peter was more reluctant to hand over the sharps?

2. What would I have done if Peter was more insistent that I call Janine, who was probably busy caring for other young people?

3. What do I say to Sienna to reassure her as well as being respectful of Peter's confidentiality?

# Reflective questions for the team

1. Could we have offered Peter the time and nurture earlier in the evening, so he felt he had someone to talk things through with, and thus avoided his self-harming behaviours?

2. How closely do we need to monitor Peter's well-being now and who is best placed to do this?

3. How should we plan further support for Peter?

4. What resources can we access to help young people cope with their difficult emotions without self-harming?

5. What support can we give team members who have helped a young person who has self-harmed?

6. How can we support each other when young people do not accept our care and therefore do not validate our identity as carers?

# CASE STUDY 6: BOHEMIA

## Background

Bohemia is a 15-year-old girl who has long blonde hair and an interest in fashion. She likes putting on different make-up and doing the other girls' hairstyles when they are getting on well together. She has opinions on the different brands of make-up and would like to become a make-up artist. She chats a lot about popular culture and knows what is happening in the lives of celebrities. She mainly goes along with activities and will have a go at most things that are happening in our house. Relationships are sometimes turbulent for Bohemia as she can be very pleasant and charming but also is known to upstage her peers or discredit or misrepresent them.

Often when there has been a disagreement among the girls in our house, Bohemia goes to her room and watches romantic comedies. She also writes long letters to her friend and boyfriend. She has only been living with us for four months and is more invested in her previous relationships. She does not believe she will be with us long and it is being discussed between our staff teams that she does not appear to be motivated to develop stronger relationships here. However, writing letters is something she spends a long time doing, especially at bedtime. She is also attempting to write a make-up blog. This is in its early stages, but we are encouraging her to experiment.

Bohemia was placed in foster care at the age of six. She spent her early years in a family where there was a lot of violence between her parents and also her two older brothers. Both of her brothers have spent time in locked facilities after community intervention did not reduce the risks to others. Following these separate periods, Bohemia's oldest brother, Lucas, committed a violent crime and is currently in prison as an adult. Bohemia is still in touch with both her brothers, who seem to hold her in very high regard. However, Bohemia can never quite be sure that they will fulfil promises. She had spent an afternoon with her mother twice a year when she was growing up, until her mother passed away last year.

Bohemia's previous foster carers, Jane and Gary, are regularly in touch with her. They really tried hard to keep Bohemia safe and did a very good job of parenting her. This cannot have been easy, but they had provided a placement for the past five years. However, towards the end of this placement, Bohemia had shown less regard for the boundaries they had put in place and had begun staying out all night without firm arrangements for her safe whereabouts. It was suspected she may have been visiting older males. Although Bohemia cannot go back to live with them, Jane and Gary have pledged to stay in touch and support Bohemia in a planned way when she leaves residential care. Bohemia is both grateful and resentful for this offer in equal measure. She is also quite jealous of the 13-year-old girl who is now in a foster placement with Jane and Gary.

# Today's events

Bohemia had her make-up spread out on the dining room table and we needed to clear up so we could get ready for tea. I was helping her tidy her things away and, to get it all through to her room quicker, I put some items into my pocket. Bohemia started shouting that I was going to take her eyelash curlers home. I put my hand on her forearm and tried to explain my true intent. She then ran to get another worker and young person, alleging that I had grabbed her.

## Questions

- How do I reassure Bohemia that I did not intend to keep her items?

- How do we deal with her allegation?

- How do we resolve this and continue with the plans for the evening?

- How do we reassure all the young people in our care?

## My practice

| | My practice | Why did I do this? |
|---|---|---|
| 1 | The two young people, my colleague Lina and I stood in the dining room. Lina calmly asked what had happened. I put the items from my pocket on the table, stood still and said nothing at this point. | I needed to regulate myself before contributing. I am aware that I am a male, and I was with three females. I am aware of my gender vulnerability and power so wanted to take a step back and consider how to approach this. |
| 2 | Bohemia was agitated and continued to say that I grabbed her. I said, *'I touched you on the arm, Bohemia, in a friendly way to show you that I meant no harm. I realise now that I should not have done that. I am sorry.'* | I decided to take ownership of my own actions and reflect openly that I could have done things differently. |
| 3 | Erin, the other young person, said, *'You can't go round touching girls, ya perv!'* The two girls linked arms with each other in defiance. I said, *'Look, what's done is done; I have put the things on the table.* [I pulled out my pocket to show I had nothing in there.] *Let's get them all put away and then we can have tea.'* | I wanted to try and de-escalate things and ignore Erin's taunts. I knew her background too and the difficulties she had had, so her response was not out of character. I didn't want to enflame the issue by defending myself as we would get locked in positions. I wanted to move us all forward. |

| | My practice | Why did I do this? |
|---|---|---|
| 4 | Bohemia said, '*We are not putting anything away for you.*' Erin looked at her and, as one, they climbed on the dining room table and stood there. Lina began putting bits of make-up in the carrycase. | I didn't touch any make-up as I thought it would escalate matters. |
| 5 | I left the room. The girls mocked, '*Run away, run away!*' | I decided to remove myself from the dining room as it was me the girls were targeting. I knew that Lina would be able to calm things down. I was within earshot if she needed anything else from me. |
| 6 | I tactically swapped with Robyn who had been playing Monopoly in the side room with William. | Perhaps another female figure to support Lina would be helpful. |
| 7 | William asked, '*What's happening? – what's going on with them?*' (meaning the girls).<br><br>I said, '*They are needing to have a bit of a chat, that's all. They are not happy, but things will all work out.*' | I didn't need to go through all of the events with William. It was not his business, and I did not want to risk him running through and becoming involved in the standoff. |
| 8 | I distracted him and we carried on playing Monopoly. Thankfully, he was content with that. | I felt a bit more useful doing something positive with William and needed to work out in my head how to respond to the allegation. The Monopoly bought me time to think and self-regulate. |
| 9 | After about half an hour everything seemed settled in the dining room. I just continued sitting with William, however, and did not go through. | William was happy that he had some one-to-one time and although I was aware that tea was now late, it wasn't essential that things needed to run to schedule. |
| 10 | Lina then came through and told us it was time for tea. The girls seemed to have moved on and were talking about a reality programme on TV and what the characters were doing and saying to each other. It was not my 'cup of tea', so I did not contribute to their conversation. I calmly and purposefully spoke with William during the meal about what he was going to do in the evening. | I also wanted to see how things were going before considering how I could repair my relationship with Bohemia. |

→

| | My practice | Why did I do this? |
|---|---|---|
| 11 | After the arrangements had been made about the evening activities, I took Lina to one side to ask if she would come and speak with Bohemia with me. | I did not want to leave it too long before speaking directly with Bohemia as I wanted her to know I cared enough to want to re-engage with her. I also wanted a witness as I did not want her to make more allegations against me. |
| 12 | Lina agreed and we took Bohemia into the 'Quiet Room'. | We did this from a point of shared understanding. We both knew that it would not be positive to have the conversation in the dining room, where the situation had happened, nor in Bohemia's bedroom as this was too intimate a room to be discussing allegations. Neither would it be sensible to have the conversation in front of other young people, from a sensitivity point of view from Bohemia's perspective, as well as a planned de-escalation perspective. Bohemia did not need an audience when we talked to her about what had happened. |
| 13 | I said, '*Bohemia, I want to apologise for any misunderstanding about your make-up stuff. I should not have put it in my pocket. I am sorry.*' | I wanted to take the adult role and talk initially about the root cause of the issue. I wanted her to hear that I took responsibility for my part in the problem. |
| 14 | She said defensively, '*You were going to take my eyelash curlers home!!*' I gently joked with her, '*I am a bloke, Bohemia! I wouldn't know what to do with eyelash curlers!*' | I thought that a bit of humour, fun at my own expense, would help lighten things. |
| 15 | She retorted, '*You wanted to give them to your girlfriend!*' I said calmly, '*Nothing like that entered my head. All I was doing was clearing up the table, taking the stuff to your room because it was teatime. I was trying to be helpful. I have said that I am sorry for putting your things in my pocket.*' | I wanted to try and say this in a neutral tone so Bohemia could see the facts. I tried not to be defensive but knew that I would have to justify my actions later, to more people. I wanted a clear picture in Lina's mind too for what had happened, as she did not see it. |

| | My practice | Why did I do this? |
|---|---|---|
| 16 | She was adamant, *'You are not sorry – and you grabbed me. I am raising a complaint about you!'* I sighed involuntarily and said, *'Of course you can raise a complaint. Lina, will you be able to support Bohemia to do this?'* | I supported her wish to make a complaint for two reasons. Firstly (from a selfish point of view), if I was seen to be trying to dissuade her then it might be perceived by others that I was guilty and, secondly, I believe that children and young people have the right to complain and be treated seriously. This helps develop trust for future situations where they may need to complain for more genuine reasons. |

## How might these theories apply to the situation?

• Need

• Attachment

• Complex and disenfranchised grief

• Drama triangle

• Transactional analysis

## How might these models of intervention apply?

• Secure base

• Cognitive behavioural therapy

• Emotional intelligence

## Reflective questions for me as a worker

1. What might have been different if I had stayed to try and persuade the girls off the table?

2. Did I speak with Bohemia afterwards at the right time, or would it have been better to do it at a different time?

3. What do I need to do from now on to protect myself?

4. Who can I chat this through with?

5. How can I further repair my relationship with Bohemia?

## Reflective questions for the team

1. How else could we have handled this?

2. What is the policy in our service for supporting workers when allegations have been made against them?

3. What are the recording requirements in our service for allegations?

4. Who else needs to be informed of the allegation and our team response?

5. What changes in practice are necessary in our team now?

6. Bohemia is likely to share the content of her complaint with Erin, William and Hannah (who was not there at the time). How can we support all four young people to make sense of this situation?

# CASE STUDY 7: JOSH

## Background

Josh is 15 and comes from a Traveller family who live in a small housing area on the edge of a larger town. The family have lived in the same house for about seven years and are very involved with their own community. Josh's older sister lives next door with her three children, who all attend the local school just across the other side of the park. Josh has been brought up with a clear sense of identity and is loyal to his family.

When Josh was 13, the family came to the attention of social work when a neighbour complained to the local authority of a smell coming from one of the outbuildings. It turned out that Josh's parents had not disposed of a dead cat effectively and the animal was in an outbuilding covered with maggots and flies. Josh's parents did not see that they needed to protect the children from this. Questions were asked and referrals made. Out-of-hours social workers had arranged on two occasions for the children to stay in the care of other family members after they had arrived and found their parents intoxicated. Social workers undertook a comprehensive assessment considering the role of the extended family in looking after Josh and his two brothers and sister. After some time, they concluded that all the children in the family had too much responsibility for their age and neither their parents nor their extended family could keep them safe. Josh's parents did not agree with what social workers were asking them to change.

Alternative care placements were found for the children, and they needed to move schools. Although they had regular time with their parents, Josh was placed separately from the other children, and he did not get to see them often. About four months after Josh was placed with his foster family, he was charged with the rape of the daughter of his foster carer. He then ran away and went missing for a month. He found his way back home, where he was harboured. He was discovered by police after a family row had escalated and spilled out onto the street. They found Josh hiding under a truck at the rear of the property with two of the family dogs. He came to our residential service from there and has been with us for around nine months. The rape charge did not proceed. His parents have come regularly to visit Josh and things have been going very well. The longer-term plan is for Josh to return home to the care of his parents when he reaches 16.

## Today's events

Today I was taking Josh for his first supervised home visit. He was really happy to be going and had increased his telephone calls home in anticipation. It had been decided that I would accompany him as we had a good relationship and I had also facilitated some family visits when his parents had come to see him. We had a tentative alliance over our discussions around Josh's needs. They wanted him to come home to live with them as soon as possible. It was a sunny afternoon, and the family were in the garden when we arrived. There were three little children playing in a sand pit and a woman with a baby, none of whom were known to me. There were four other adults present, including Josh's parents, and all of them were openly smoking cannabis and clearly stoned.

## Questions

- Should the visit go ahead?
- What are the risks involved?
- What responsibility do I have to the other children present?
- What are the protective factors?
- What do I need to do to keep myself safe?

## My practice

|  | My practice | Why did I do this? |
|---|---|---|
| 1 | I saw Josh look at me a bit nervously. He knew what was happening and wasn't sure what I would do.<br><br>I decided to stay and see how things developed. | Josh was looking forward to his visit and might be upset if we left. However, I was aware of the legal implications of his family's actions. I was not prepared for this.<br><br>I considered we still had time to leave if I felt Josh was at risk at any point. I thought I could justify my decision to others but would keep this open to change. |
| 2 | I said to Josh quietly, '*We will see how this goes but you need to stay where I can see you. You want "people" to be able to say you made good decisions today.*' | I was worried that I was now complicit in allowing Josh to be present while people were under the influence of cannabis. I realised that Josh was 15 years old and had most likely been around his family in the past under the same circumstances. I wanted him to know that he was responsible for his own actions but that I was still taking the adult role. |
| 3 | Josh eyed me with uncertainty. He went to play with the children in the sand pit. From this vantage point he could orient himself to what was going on. I smiled at people and went to speak directly with Josh's mum. She did not get up. | I wanted to carry on as if everything was normal, although I was annoyed with the family for putting Josh in this position. They knew he was coming for his first supervised home visit and how much he was looking forward to it. And they must have known there would be implications. I figured that I could deal with my relationship with them, and the assessment of other people later. If everyone was safe we could carry on. |

| | My practice | Why did I do this? |
|---|---|---|
| 4 | I sat on a garden chair near Josh. | I wanted him to enjoy the visit without me seeming nervous. |
| 5 | It looked like they were staying in the garden for the afternoon, but I figured I would stay there if people went inside. | I did not want to expose myself to more fumes than was necessary as I needed to drive back safely. |
| 6 | I asked Josh's mum to introduce me to everyone and she did. I hastily rehearsed their names in my head so I could recall them. At the first opportunity I would need to write them down. I thought I might take a note on my phone when I get a chance. | Remembering everyone's names might be important later. I could justify taking a note under the circumstances. |
| 7 | Josh began interacting well with the people around him. He joked with his dad and some of the other adults. He was kind to the children. I stayed quite quiet. | I felt a bit out of my comfort zone and wanted to end the visit. Nothing unsafe was going on though and although I would have had justification, I thought I would just observe. |
| 8 | I texted my manager to let him know the situation on the visit. He advised to just keep assessing the risks and do what I thought was best. | I thought I had better keep him informed so that everything was transparent and I was not alone in making the decisions. |
| 9 | After about half an hour or so, Josh said to me, 'Cally needs a drink.' I said, 'Come straight back' and he went inside. I followed him to the kitchen door almost immediately. He looked at me like he was a bit confused. | Although I did not want to chaperone Josh that closely, I thought that I would protect him by keeping him in sight, so he could not later be accused of anything. I was not sure if there was alcohol in the house or if he might access any substances. |
| 10 | I had a good look in the kitchen as Josh made Cally and himself some orange juice. The kitchen was mostly clean and tidy. Nothing of any concern. | I was conscious that I was there to support and supervise Josh, not anyone else. However, I could not ignore the needs of the other children. |

→

| | My practice | Why did I do this? |
|---|---|---|
| 11 | Josh came outside and sat on the grass beside the chair I had claimed. Another 20 minutes or so passed and then Josh asked if he could go and see Cally's rabbit. This was in a garden a couple of houses down the street. I said that he had come to spend time with his mum and dad and suggested that he go and sit beside his mum for a chat. | I wanted him to get the most he could out of the visit, and I had not seen them interact much. |
| 12 | Josh said, 'She's baked. I want to see the rabbit. I haven't seen it before, and I like rabbits.' I agreed to this but said I would come with him. | I thought I would be led by him if that was what he wanted. I probably would have let him under other circumstances as well. |
| 13 | They played with the rabbit out of his hutch for a while. It looked well cared for and had a clean cage.<br><br>When they looked like they were getting bored I said, 'We will have to go now, Josh. Let's go and say goodbye to your mum and dad and everyone.' | I thought we had been there long enough and although it was slightly shorter than planned, nothing had gone really wrong. I thought it was a suitable time to make an exit so that it could stay that way. |
| 14 | We took Cally back to the family in the garden and I waited by the gate while Josh said goodbye. I watched him closely and waved at his dad and the woman with the baby. They all stayed where they were. | I watched from the gate because I didn't want the family to pick up that I was annoyed with them for not paying Josh enough attention. That visit was supposed to be for him, and his family blatantly smoking cannabis on a planned visit might set back the process of him going back to live at home. I knew how much he wanted this. I needed to stay calm and get us home safely. |

| My practice | Why did I do this? |
|---|---|
| Josh came away as if he was quite comfortable with everything. He had behaved well and did not give me cause for concern. | I also watched closely to see if anyone slipped anything into Josh's hand or pocket. It would not be good if Josh decided to take back substances to share with his peers in the residential house, and I needed to protect them (and myself, as I could be accused of being complicit in this). I resolved to work out in the car with him how we could be sure that there could be no 'misunderstandings' about substances entering the house, just in case I had not seen everything. I thought I had his trust, as far as I could have done, so I could work with him to keep everyone safe. |

## How might these theories apply to the situation?

• Emotional intelligence

• Labelling

• Stigma

## How might these models of intervention apply?

• De-escalation

• Opportunity-led practice

• Values-based conversations

• Harm reduction

## Reflective questions for me as a worker

1. What precedent was I setting allowing the visit to go ahead?

2. What are the pressures for Josh in this situation?

3. How can we understand this situation through a cultural lens?

4. What conversation would I need to have on the way home with Josh?

5. Who else would I need to share this information with?

6. What could I have done differently?

7. If Josh was a different age, would that have made a difference in my decision making?

## Reflective questions for the team

1. How must it feel to be removed from everything you know to a place full of strangers?

2. What do all members of our team need to know about Josh's Traveller background that would help us care effectively for him?

3. What would be the best practice in another situation where it was clear that other types of drugs had been taken by family members when we arrive for a supervised home visit?

4. Do we all know how to recognise the effects on people of different types of drugs?

# CASE STUDY 8: SORRELL

## Background

Sorrell is ten years old and the youngest of four children. She enjoys feeding the chickens and brushing Monty the pony. She likes going for walks in the woods and throwing sticks over the bridge into the water to watch them come out the other side. She could do this for hours.

Sorrell was born in a city and her life experiences outside school were somewhat limited to going to the local shop and buying crisps and newspapers. She had spent a disproportionate time for her age indoors in a very sparse home environment. Her family life had been considered chaotic with the front door being continually unlocked and people coming and going from the house, a lack of family routines and intermittent levels of care for the children. Both her parents had periodically taken heroin and all the children had spent time being cared for by their grandmother. Sorrell's oldest sister had also recently become addicted to heroin.

Sorrell cannot read or write, despite having had one-on-one support in school. She only attended three mornings a week when she lived at home as this was all she could manage. She had been regularly assessed by school psychologists and support strategies had been devised. Sorrell had been found three times in the school toilets smearing faeces on the walls.

Sorrell's older brother made an allegation that a family member had sexually assaulted him and another of his sisters. During the investigation a quantity of pornographic images had been seized from the possession of their father and the family member accused. To date, Sorrell's father is not known to have shown any remorse and continued to deny the images were his. (Sorrell knew this because her mother had told her, and she had also informed care workers on the telephone.) However, Sorrell's father and the family member are currently awaiting trial. It is unknown at this point whether or not Sorrell had been subjected to any abuse. She has not disclosed anything although she can at times use inappropriate sexualised language.

Sorrell has been in our care for about ten months and has really settled in. Country life suits her. Prior to this she had spent a week in a foster care placement before it was assessed as unsuitable for her needs. Her academic learning in our care is delivered by following a curriculum in the house, as she cannot yet emotionally manage to transition back and forth to a school classroom setting. Sorrell is assessed to be functioning at around age six to seven years old. We pride ourselves on the therapeutic work that our animals can provide for children and young people. We have staff who oversee the teaching, and all learning is offered through the core relationships Sorrell has made with workers. Her favourite worker is Harry, who is teaching her how to play the guitar.

## Today's events

Sorrell came in from the garden with Jane (a care worker). Sorrell was carrying a container of strawberries that had been grown in the polytunnel. Sorrell was happy that she had picked them, and she told me that the white ones left behind would turn red tomorrow. Suddenly a wailing sound could be heard from upstairs. Trent (aged nine) had discovered his new watch was missing. He came dashing downstairs, followed by Samuel (a care worker). Sorrell started pushing over chairs and throwing table mats. The strawberries went everywhere. It was clear she was wearing the watch. Because of the disruption it took a few minutes for Trent to become aware that Sorrell had his watch.

## Questions

- How do we restore calm?

- How do we support Trent?

- How do we work to get Sorrell to give the watch back?

- How do we teach Sorrell that she can't take other people's things?

## My practice

| | My practice | Why did I do this? |
|---|---|---|
| 1 | Jane and I encouraged Sorrell away from Trent. Samuel encouraged Trent through to the conservatory with assurances that he would have his watch returned. | We needed to separate the children so we could deal with their needs individually and de-escalate the situation. |
| 2 | Jane and I stayed close to Sorrell as she ran out into the garden. She went to sit on the bench and swung her legs vigorously. Jane and I sat either side of her. We stayed calm but ready to move again if she got up and ran. | We needed to ensure Sorrell was safe and to give her time to self-regulate. |
| 3 | Sorrell was still clearly full of adrenaline. She said tensely, *'It's my watch, not his.'* I said, *'It looks very nice. Can I see it?'* | Although we knew that it was not hers, Jane and I also knew that she needed to be calmer before we could address the issue. I wanted to get a closer look at the item and to let Sorrell feel we could support her without judgement. |

| | My practice | Why did I do this? |
|---|---|---|
| 4 | Sorrell pulled up her sleeve a tiny bit and put it straight back down again. I got a glimpse. Jane asked, *'Where did you get it?'* I tried to keep my body relaxed. I took a focused breath softly out and in. | I thought this might be too direct, too soon, and Sorrell might run off. I didn't want her to pick up on my tension. |
| 5 | She said, *'I got it from my mum at the weekend.'* Her mum had visited. I said, *'Your mum had a good time here, didn't she? Could you imagine how lucky she was to see that toad up at the Mabie woods? I think he knew she was coming and popped out to say hello!'* | I wanted to be less direct and for Sorrell to be calmer before we tackled the issue of theft. I thought of the 'shield of shame' (Golding and Hughes, 2012 on p. 114), where she might minimise, deny, blame others and become angry. I didn't want her experience of shame to get in the way of her acceptance of wrongdoing and make it harder for her to make different choices in the future. |
| 6 | I suggested, *'Why don't we go for a walk up there now to see if we can find him?'* | This way we could use movement to help the adrenaline to dissipate and we could all relax. We could trust that Trent was safely with other workers, and we could have an eye on where the watch was to also keep it safe. |
| 7 | We walked up to the Mabie woods and chatted about other things on the way: things that Sorrell knew about the trees and the birds that lived there. This took about half an hour. | This could have facilitated a sense of control and mastery for Sorrell. It was calming for us all. |
| 8 | Sorrell picked up a stick and began poking a hole at the base of a tree. She was going deeper and deeper in. She was doing no real harm, but I took the opportunity to see if she would hand the watch over. *'That looks a bit dirty in that rabbit hole, Sorrell. I tell you what, why don't you pass me the watch for safekeeping, just to make sure it doesn't get broken or scratched. It is a very nice watch.'* | I said 'the' watch rather than 'your' watch, as I did not want to validate her construction of the story.<br><br>I did want to validate the conversation we had earlier though, that we all agreed it was a nice watch. |

| | **My practice** | **Why did I do this?** |
|---|---|---|
| 9 | Sorrell agreed and handed over the watch, which I put in my pocket. | I had helped her not to 'lose face' but had given her the opportunity to make a good choice. Leaving her with choice was important, I thought. |
| 10 | I nodded to Jane as Sorrell continued to play. I wandered away from them and called back to the house by phone. I updated Samuel and said I would return with the watch. | We needed to communicate as a staff team. This would have been expected between us. We made a plan to return the watch and keep the children separate for the rest of the afternoon until a conversation could be had with Sorrell. This would hopefully avoid other issues or quarrelling. |
| 11 | I excused myself to go and *'put the kettle on'*. Jane and I could anticipate each other's part, and Jane said she and Sorrell would be another 15 minutes or so as they had *'not quite finished playing'*. | Sorrell thought she was getting more time in the woods, which she loved. |
| 12 | After we had had juice and a snack, Jane and I sat on the conservatory sofas with Sorrell in the late afternoon sun. I said, *'You know, Sorrell, that watch is very like the one belonging to Trent.'* She said, *'It's mine.'* I responded gently, *'I don't remember your mum giving you a watch at the weekend. I am wondering if you would have really liked her to give you one in real life.'* She dropped her eyes. *'It's mine.'* Jane said, *'It is so nice. If it was yours and somebody else took it, do you think you might be mad at them?'* Sorrell said, *'I would be super-crazy and smash them to pieces!'* Jane said, *'I am wondering if that was the way Trent was feeling earlier when he found his watch was gone.'* | We had decided to work together to address the issue when the household was relaxed and the other two children were occupied elsewhere.

We needed to find a non-shaming way to help Sorrell learn. |

| | My practice | Why did I do this? |
|---|---|---|
| 13 | I said, *'People like their special things, don't they? I like this necklace that I got on holiday. I think I would be upset too if someone took it. Trent needs to get his watch back. I wonder if we can agree with everyone that people leave other people's things and don't take them away. Then we can be sure that nobody is taking your special things either.'* | I didn't say to her that Trent already had his watch back as this might enrage her at this point. I wanted her to feel that she was part of the discussion as it was worked through, at a pace she could process effectively. I felt a bit dishonest but thought that I was attuned to Sorrell's age and stage of development. I tried not to be accusing, more to appeal to her natural child's self-centredness. |
| 14 | Jane said, *'Yes, I agree with this. I like my watch too and want to keep it safe.'* I said, *'Of course, if someone wants to lend their special thing to someone for a time, that is a bit different. I think we need to discuss that with everyone, so we are all clear.'* | Jane played along to align with Sorrell's presenting age and understanding.<br><br>I knew how confusing and messy this could all get, so was keen to discuss this with all three children in the household later to support their development. Although draining for us as workers, this situation was a gift as an opportunity to help guide the children in a safe environment. |

## How might these theories apply to the situation?

• (Loss of the) assumptive world

• Moral development

• Need

• Mastery

• Neurosequential model

## How might these models of intervention apply?

• Trauma-sensitive practice

• Mentalisation (how might the other person be feeling/thinking)

• Mediation

## Reflective questions for me as a worker

1. Should I have left Jane to deal with this on her own as she has a better relationship with Sorrell?

2. What else could I have done to de-escalate the situation and achieve positive outcomes?

3. What would I have done if I had been supporting Trent?

4. What do I need to think about in preparation for a discussion with all children?

## Reflective questions for the team

1. What were the possible drivers for Sorrell's behaviour and how do we support her development?

2. How would this have worked if it was a different young person?

3. How do we facilitate a conversation between Sorrell and Trent?

4. How will we plan as a team to work with all the children if this happens again?

5. How will we share this information with others?

**The following list might start to help us understand individual children's needs around stealing.**

## What motivates a young person to steal?

- Poor impulse control – wants gratification.

- A trophy.

- A positive memory – a souvenir.

- They want adult attention.

- The young person has not learned that stealing is wrong.

- They have observed other people take things that don't belong to them.

- Emotional neglect – the stolen object fills an emotional void.

- Unmet need for physical care – survival thinking and resourcefulness.

- Entitlement due to unmet physical or emotional need.

- Fear of not having enough – or of running out (could be of running out of love or stability).

- Craving what others have materially, or could also be jealousy and craving the love or status that others have.

- Expressing displaced feelings of anxiety, anger or alienation resulting from major life changes.

- Retaliation – wanting revenge for the pain that others inflicted upon them.

- Wanting to appear bold, tough and important.

- Desire to fit in with the peer group.

- Wanting to have the same identity as the person they have stolen from.

- Enjoying the thrill that comes from stealing.

- Rebelling against authority.

- Stealing items or money to buy drugs.

- Stealing to give the items to someone else to buy their affection and attention.

**What other drivers for stealing behaviours would you add?**

**What practice approaches are needed in response to the different behavioural drivers?**

# CASE STUDY 9: HAKIM

## Background

Hakim is a 13-year-old boy who enjoys playing with Lego and other construction games. He takes his creations apart and reassembles them many times over. He is not fond of other young people and much prefers his own company. He can often be found sitting talking to himself while deeply focused on what he is doing. He appears to self-soothe by going into a 'world of his own'.

He is very keen on learning from books and can be demanding of workers to sit with him and go over the schoolwork provided by his teachers at his request. He wants to do this on his own terms, often at times that are inconvenient to workers and other young people. Hakim appears to have limited regard for their points of view and can get angry if there is a delay in meeting his requests for support.

Hakim, his brother and their mother are asylum seekers. Their father is living in their country of origin with extended family and works in the X-ray department of the local hospital. Hakim's family value education, and Hakim and his brother were promptly enrolled in a school when they arrived in this country. It quickly became apparent that neither brother could manage the emotional demands of secondary school and found changing classes especially distressing. Hakim had frequently lashed out at other pupils and teachers and did not manage to attend very long before the school had concluded that this was not the right environment for him. He had also been violent to his mother and brother, hitting them both with a broom handle and an electric extension cable. Hakim also had scars on his own body from violence he had been subjected to in the community in his country of origin. He was assessed as requiring therapeutic care alongside education.

Hakim has lived with us for seven months. At first, he had taken his bed covers onto the floor and slept in the corner of his room. We had worked with other professionals to provide sensitive and trauma-informed care. Slowly, Hakim decided that he would sleep on the bed. He also had difficulty sitting still at the table to eat and would previously hover at the side of the group at the start of mealtimes, sometimes getting agitated and usually requiring attention from workers. He can manage to sit down and wait for the meal to be served now but we think he has more general sensory difficulties.

## Today's events

It had been planned that our other three other young people, Scott, Ian and Jamila, would go out to do some orienteering with workers. Hakim wanted to stay in the house and for Amanda (care worker) to do his English homework with him. Amanda, however, was also intending to support the orienteering group. Hakim realised this just before lunchtime and had become anxious. He kept repeating, *'my rights, my rights'*. Amanda had reassured him that she would help him before she went. However, through lunch he kept asking what time his *'schoolwork'* would start. Scott was irritated by Hakim and told him that he was *'not the boss of Amanda'*. Ian sided with Scott and pinged a pea, which hit Hakim on the head. Hakim must have believed Scott had done this as he rushed round and pushed Scott off his chair. He then stood over Amanda in an intimidating way tugging on her arm. Ian threw the whole of the rest of his meal at Hakim, who shouted, *'I'm telling legal meeting!'* He pushed Ian backwards and ran to his room, chased by Scott and quickly followed by me and Ricky (care worker).

## Questions

- How do we restore calm?
- How do we help Hakim manage his anxiety and controlling behaviours?
- How do we continue with the planned activities?
- How do we, as a team, support Amanda?

## My practice

| | My practice | Why did I do this? |
|---|---|---|
| 1 | Scott was pounding on Hakim's door and Hakim was attempting to hold it shut to protect himself. Ricky and I encouraged Scott away. I validated Scott's position by agreeing that he had been the wronged party. | I hoped this acknowledgement would help de-escalate the situation. |
| 2 | Although it took several minutes, Scott did leave Hakim's door. He shouted threats to harm him in the future, but Ricky managed to encourage him through into the other room. | Safety first! We needed to separate the boys so we could de-escalate things further. |
| 3 | I went into Hakim's room. He was pacing around jabbing the air with his fist and talking to himself. | I wanted to risk assess his presentation but also keep myself safe. While Hakim was pacing around, I kept near the door so I could leave quickly if needed. I spoke slowly and calmly so that he could use me to co-regulate. |
| 4 | Hakim knew I was there as I continued to talk. I talked about the things I could see in his room. | I wanted to find concrete things that I could help Hakim anchor his awareness to. |

| | My practice | Why did I do this? |
|---|---|---|
| 5 | After several minutes, Hakim appeared to be less agitated. I still stayed physically back from him although he had stopped punching the air. | I realised that he may still have adrenaline in his system and if he perceived me to be too close, he might have lashed out. |
| 6 | Hakim was worried that Amanda was going out and, for some time, I negotiated with him to stay in his room while I went to find Amanda. | I did not want to risk him coming into contact with the other young people while he may still be highly anxious as this may trigger another incident. They would all have still been adrenalised too. |
| 7 | Amanda and I discussed how to approach things. She wanted to go and do the English home-work with Hakim and then go out with the other young people as planned. I was in two minds, as Hakim had just controlled the whole situation and placed others in a state of alarm. (No one was hurt.)<br><br>Although I was uncomfortable with 'rewarding' Hakim with his desired outcome (Amanda's attention) after his aggressive behaviour, I agreed to stay with Ian and Jamila while she went to speak with Hakim. | Amanda had thought that this would give her a chance to speak with Hakim about his behaviours as well as meet the needs of the other young people.<br><br>I could have swapped with Amanda's plans for the whole afternoon. She could have stayed in the house with Hakim and I could have gone orienteering, but it seemed to us both that we should stay with the firm plans as made.<br><br>Also, we needed to reduce the risks by giving Hakim the time as planned. Another incident would delay the after-noon for the other young people, who would miss out and resent Hakim for this. Four young people together in the house after this incident may increase risk. |
| 8 | Jamila was deciding what to wear for her orienteering experience. She asked if Hakim was going to be *punished for pushing everyone*. I told her that he would be spoken with, and things would be dealt with prop-erly. I focused our discussion on the shoes that might be appro-priate to wear for the outing. | I did not want to get into conversations with Jamila about how any situation with another young person would be handled. I believed she had the right to expect justice for peers and herself (albeit she was not involved in this issue). We can never be sure what young people have experienced in their lives and I could never have anticipated the ways in which she may have been triggered by what she had witnessed. So, I thought that my answer was balanced and fair but not minimising. |

| | My practice | Why did I do this? |
|---|---|---|
| 9 | Ian and Scott were also getting ready to go. They had both calmed down as time had moved on. Ricky had helped them regulate but now Scott could not find his coat and was getting agitated again. I stayed with Jamila rather than helping support Ricky to look for the coat. | I did not want Jamila to follow me along the bedroom corridor where Scott was. I wanted to minimise confusion and stay as a reliable adult alongside Jamila. She was quieter than the boys but that did not mean that she did not need attention. I thought Ricky was managing to help Scott. |
| 10 | Amanda had finished the English homework support with Hakim and again had persuaded him to stay in his room. She and I exchanged glances and I said to Jamila, 'I'm going to speak with Hakim again. I hope you have a lovely time. Drink lots of water and take photos! See you when you get back.' | Amanda and I knew that it would be best for Hakim to have someone with him until the other young people had left the house. They were still buzzing about getting ready. I could rely on Amanda to take over as the adult support to Jamila and facilitate their plans and she could rely on me to take over the adult role with Hakim. |
| 11 | Hakim was playing Lego in his room. He seemed content. I asked him how he had got on with his schoolwork. | I did not know what Amanda had said to Hakim about the incident and did not want to start further discussions about this until at least the group had left the house in case this triggered any outbursts. I did know that Hakim strongly believes that he is entitled to an education. Asking him about it could be the start of a positive conversation. |
| 12 | Hakim did not answer but I gently sat down beside him on the floor. | Hakim understands more English than he can speak but I did not press him to engage with me if he chose not to. I tried to be friendly by sitting near him to give him the opportunity, and so that he could have some of his attachment needs met. If there was no adult nearby providing attention, he may have felt abandoned, especially if Amanda was going out. |

| | My practice | Why did I do this? |
|---|---|---|
| 13 | I waited for a bit, and he began speaking about what he was doing with the Lego. He did not raise the subject of the incident with me. I decided to play with Lego for a short while after the group went out, then withdraw so he could play alone. | I considered that there would be time to discuss his behaviour later when there were two workers present. It would better protect both of us to have a witness present.<br><br>I was happy to leave it just now unless Hakim raised anything. As a staff team we could take a planned approach to addressing his behaviour. |

## How might these theories apply to the situation?

• Assumptive world

• Neurosequential model

• Power

• Locus of control

• Need

• Systems

## How might these models of intervention apply?

• Transactional analysis

• Behaviour chain analysis

• Group work

## Reflective questions for me as a worker

1. How emotionally intelligent was my interaction with each young person?

2. What else could I have done to offer a secure base to the young people?

3. How else could I have supported Amanda?

4. While the group are out, what can I do to plan for a calm evening on their return?

## Reflective questions for the team

1. What will be our team approach to the discussion we will need to have with Hakim about his behaviour?

2. Do we need to discuss the possible drivers for Hakim's behaviour and any additional management strategies with anyone else?

3. How will we set boundaries for Hakim that support his learning in a predictable and consistent ways?

4. How can we promote physical and psychological safety for all young people in our care?

5. How can we support each other, bearing in mind we can never know what previous experiences our colleagues have had and what they might find triggering?

# CASE STUDY 10: POPPY

## Background

Poppy is a 15-year-old girl with a great sense of humour and a mischievous laugh. She likes to do scrapbooking, painting and journaling. She has had a good education for her age, and she attends the local college to learn to cook. Her ambition is to become a chef in London. She loves food but does not enjoy physical activity and is overweight.

When Poppy likes someone she is 'all-in', although she struggles to keep friends very long. She is often considered manipulative by other young people, and some care workers find her very difficult to manage. Other workers feel sorry for her and try to help her as best they can by giving her time and attention.

Poppy's mum had some mental health difficulties. Poppy clearly had no control over this, and it has affected her whole life to date. As an infant, Poppy was delayed from walking due to her mother keeping her for long periods in a baby buggy. When Poppy was little, her mum took her to the doctor regularly for checks. It was a very long while before this situation was named as a suspected fabrication of symptoms. Poppy was nine when she came into foster care with a same-sex (female) couple, Mia and Jade. They ran a high-end seafood restaurant in a picturesque tourist destination village by the sea. They lived in the flat above the restaurant and saw that Poppy did not want for anything materially. Initially the arrangement worked well as they could both be there for Poppy after school. Her homework was always done, and they went on nice trips together. The agreement with the fostering agency was that one adult would be in the flat with Poppy each night, but as time went on, they both spent time in the restaurant while Poppy was regularly left alone.

Poppy spent a lot of time online and when she became a teenager she started going on dating sites. She made herself very vulnerable by posting nude pictures of herself and befriending older males. Child protection services were involved, and safety planning put in place around her supervision and access to the internet. Around the same time, circumstances beyond anyone's control meant that the couple had to close the restaurant. Their marriage subsequently broke down and they held Poppy responsible for this. By mutual agreement between the agency, Mia and Jade, they deregistered as carers. Poppy went to another foster carer and began running away. She was 14 when she came into our care in a residential house with four other young people. She has been with us just over a year.

## Today's events

Poppy's mum had visited yesterday, and Poppy found it difficult to sleep last night. She had eaten all the sweets that her mum had brought all at once in front of a worker, who spent a great deal of time during the evening listening to Poppy's difficulties with her mum. These were difficulties that anyone would have a hard time coming to terms with. I was not there yesterday, but I was later told about the events by another worker, who was not happy Poppy had been allowed to eat all the sweets.

Poppy had a couple of disagreements with other young people today, and as a staff team we had worked hard to keep the group occupied and engaged in activities. It was Jake's birthday, and we had a special tea and a birthday cake for him. Poppy joined in. Later, when Lucas came in from football training, he opened the ice cream. Straight away, Poppy piled a bowl very high for herself too. I thought this was excessive given all that she had eaten in the last 24 hours.

## Questions

- Do I need to do anything?

- If I decide to do something, how do I effectively offer care without shaming Poppy?

- How do I support my co-workers who are concerned about Poppy's behaviours?

- How do I challenge Poppy without outwardly undermining other workers?

- How do I stay relaxed with the other young people who do not have the same issues with food as Poppy does?

# My practice

| | My practice | Why did I do this? |
|---|---|---|
| 1 | I did decide to intervene. | I agreed with the rationale of the worker who was not happy about Poppy eating all the sweets. I would like to do my best to care for her even if this means I won't be popular with her. |
| 2 | I said quietly and gently to her, *'Poppy, that seems like quite a lot in one bowl. Why don't you pop half in this bowl, and I can put it in the freezer for you to have tomorrow?'* | I didn't want to draw attention to her behaviours in front of other people in case she felt ashamed. I did not think that I should say that she should have none at all because I did not want her to perceive me as punitive. I decided to go for a harm-minimising approach. |
| 3 | Poppy looked horrified. She became agitated and said, *'No, why should I?'*<br><br>I responded gently, *'Well, you know, you have had cake and treats yesterday and today, and we all need to keep healthy diets.'* | I needed to be clear why I was saying this, and I had already started down this path so needed to give her respectful reasons. |

| | My practice | Why did I do this? |
|---|---|---|
| 4 | Poppy immediately threw the plate at the wall, and it smashed. She screamed, '*I hate you – you old ratty cow face!*' and stormed off to her bedroom. I signalled with my eyes to my co-worker Max asking him to go to her room and speak with her. | I did not take offence as I realised that this was Poppy's response to being triggered.<br><br>I knew Poppy was likely to be in tears but if I went through to speak with her, I might make things worse and she might start throwing items around. I decided it was best to clear up the ice cream and broken plate and give her some time. I was sure that Max could help her regulate as I have worked with him a lot and know his temperament and values. |
| 5 | Robbie, another young person, came into the kitchen and asked, '*What's wrong with her?*'<br><br>I said, '*She just needs a minute or so.*' He said, '*She better not be spoiling people's birthdays, or I will stab her.*' I asked him not to talk like that as it would make everyone get '*uptight*'. I asked him to '*go have a laugh with the others and tell them about what had happened earlier when Max nearly fell in the pond*'. | I did not get into any details with Robbie, as it was none of his business. I wanted to keep my emotions well regulated. I knew there was no real risk of Poppy being stabbed and it was just a figure of speech Robbie used.<br><br>I wanted to de-escalate the situation and redirect the conversation. I needed to be the adult. |
| 6 | After a few minutes and when I could see that the others were engaged in conversation with another worker, I went through to Poppy's room. I knocked on the door, which was already open, and I could see her. '*Can I come in?*' | I didn't want to leave it too long as Poppy might feel a sense of rejection that I was not bothered about how she felt. I realised that she had experienced abandonment previously and the incident may be triggering her in many ways. I wanted to show I cared. |
| 7 | She was still crying. She shouted, '*No!*' but Max said, '*Yes of course, me and Poppy were just having a chat.*' Poppy said, '*I hate you – you called me fat!*' She carried on crying. I said, '*Poppy, I didn't say that. I just suggested that a smaller portion would be a healthier option. I would say the same to myself.*' | I wanted to be calm, clear and realistic. I wanted to be the adult. |

→

| | My practice | Why did I do this? |
|---|---|---|
| 8 | She was adamant, *'You called me fat because I was eating too much.'* I responded, *'I said that you could put half the bowlful in the freezer for tomorrow. I didn't say you were eating too much. And I only said that because I care what happens to you. When we have sugar it affects our mood – it spikes and then dips. I know you have had a tough time over the past couple of days and I was wanting to help you stay calm and get through the night without any issues. I know you didn't see it that way, so I am sorry.'* | I didn't want to get into all the other reasons why it was not a good idea for Poppy to gorge on food. I wanted to appeal to her self-interest in the 'here and now' and let her know that her difficult emotions had been acknowledged. She knows workers speak with each other so would hopefully know that the whole team were aware of her needs. |
| 9 | Poppy looked down sulkily. Max added, *'You see, Poppy, this was what I was meaning the other day. You have to separate out intent and impact – people might not intend to hurt you, but you might take it to heart and over-react.'* I stayed quiet. | I was respectful that Max was trying to be supportive and use this as a teaching moment. He was also helping to smooth things and help us repair our relationship after it had ruptured. I wanted to give Poppy a bit of time to reflect and regulate. |
| 10 | Poppy said, *'So if you care so much, why did you not say to Jordan to have half a bowl. You are still a cow face!'*<br><br>I ignored the insult and said, *'He needs a different sort of care. You all do. We are all different. There are limits for us all. He didn't have as much in his bowl for one thing, and I know that you have had lots of sugary foods recently. I would put a limit on me too. It's all about the balance.'* There was some more small talk. | I didn't say anything about Jordan just having done physical exercise or refer to him having a different physique as that would have just taken the conversation to a different and less helpful point. |

| | My practice | Why did I do this? |
|---|---|---|
| 11 | Poppy then said, '*I actually hate you, you know!*' She had stopped crying though. I said, '*I hear you, but I know we have got along fine in the past and I don't hate you. I am looking forward to spending time doing some decoupage with you on Sunday if you would still like to. I have always wanted to try that.*' | I could have kept going trying to get us back on track but if I had kept on trying to justify my actions, we would have gone round in circles, and I had already made my point.<br><br>I wanted to get the conversation away from food. |
| 12 | Max looked baffled. I brought out a craft magazine cutting from my pocket that I had looked out for to show Poppy. '*I was going to show you this tonight.*' She looked at it for a bit.<br><br>I said, '*I will leave you to tell Max all about the art of decoupage.*' I smiled and left her with the magazine cutting. She was a bit calmer although still not happy. | I knew that Max could have more of a grounding conversation when I left – as I was still a likely trigger for Poppy. Hopefully she would become more regulated before she re-joined the others.<br><br>Also, leaving something behind that was a sort of 'peace offering' might have helped our relationship. I wanted to be the adult doing the repair and with Poppy's attachment difficulties this hopefully left her with the knowledge that I had been previously keeping her in mind. |

## How might these theories apply to the situation?

• Attachment

• Social learning theory

• Transactional analysis

• Stigma

• Self-efficacy

• Emotional intelligence

## How might these models of intervention apply?

• Life-space interview

• Conflict management

• Opportunity-led practice

# Reflective questions for me as a worker

1. Did I need to try and guide Poppy from overeating?

2. What will I need to prepare for a debrief with the rest of my team?

3. Could my timing have been better?

4. What part does my gender (female) play in this situation alongside Max (male)?

5. What could I have done differently?

# Reflective questions for the team

1. What function might Poppy's behaviour with food serve?

2. Why should we not make assumptions about what function her behaviour serves?

3. How might Poppy's background have contributed to how she sees the world today?

4. Why is it important for us to work consistently with Poppy and do what we say we will do?

5. What team approach will we take with Poppy from this point on?

6. What team approach will we take with all of the young people?

# A LITTLE THING CALLED LOVE

It can seldom be argued that to grow into healthy functional adults, children need to feel loved. We have come a long way in this century in terms of how we respond to children who violate the behavioural boundaries that our society has set. No longer does society (in the UK) accept that physically beating children for their wrongdoings will result in behaviours that we approve of. Around us there is also every indication that shaming children does not do much long-term good either. We continue to pursue, at national and local policy levels, evidence-based ways of responding to the circumstances and behaviours of children and their families that result in the need for children to enter public care. And there continues to be a most welcome (UK national) challenge to improve the care experience of children and young people.

It seems fitting to round this book up with some thoughts on practical ways we could develop the culture in which love in the 'care system' is possible so children can be gifted the foundations on which to thrive and contribute to shaping a different future.

In effect, love cannot be anything other than an individualised construct. Yet those who are in professional caregiving roles may be left confused without clear guidance and leadership on boundaries and the way concepts around love should be approached in their care setting.

Firstly, language needs to be carefully considered. As the word 'love' means different things to different people, professional caregivers must think through the impact of the overt use of the word in their unique contexts. Some of our children in care may have previously experienced the word expressed in flippant, empty or abusive ways. If the child does not already have a solid basis on which to experience the word 'love' in the care environment, the caregiver may be unwittingly retraumatising them by saying it.

Some of our children in care may have experienced the word 'love' in sexually abusive or coercive contexts in the past and misinterpret the intent of a caregiver. This may bring allegations, confusion, mistrust and rupture to the relationship, which may manifest in subtle yet complex ways. Importantly, the caregiver may not know the child's background, and the child themselves may not understand how and why they have been triggered.

There could also be unintended consequences if a child experiences the caregiver's expression of the word 'love' as 'commitment' or 'investment', Why then does the placement end and why are they sent away? As they start to find the capacity to love (if we are connecting this word with trust), it must be truly awful to be rewarded with disconnection, abandonment and an 'exit strategy': a rejection amplified because they dared to invest.

# Transitions

It is imperative that we use what we know about the needs of individual children to support the development of trust and psychological safety when children need to move placement, even if this takes a bit longer than budget holders are at first comfortable with. (To begin to change care cultures in this respect, we need to get better at evidencing the impact on the public purse of actions in one system impacting positively or negatively on another.) We need to use the available evidence base (observation and listening + research) to figure out the best possible ways to love and support when children move to other care provision. Additionally, we must fully consider policy on the ongoing support and facilitation of relationships that matter.

Thinking about the words we use to foster emotionally and psychologically safe relationships, practitioners need to increase their vocabulary to further define love in context. For example, they may need to reflect on themes of forgiveness, tolerance, trust, empathy, being attuned, acceptance, unconditional positive regard or working to reduce possibilities of a child experiencing misplaced shame. If we decide to tell a child we love them, then this reflection in advance is vital.

Actions also speak louder than words, so it may not even be necessary to articulate or define love in any such subjective terms. A child who is cared for as an individual within group care, where their personal uniqueness is taken into account, and where caregivers hold them in mind when making decisions, will *feel* a sense that they matter and are important. A care culture where the basic care is excellent, for example where every child can be sure that their preferences and eccentricities around food will be accommodated and nurtured willingly, where adults go out of their way to invest time in young people, where their aspirations and potential are valued, could be considered a culture of love.

Love could also mean being sorry. And... the big one: love could mean taking responsibility in the relationship as the regulating adult. This might include owning our part in a relationship rupture, validating the impact and attempting to repair the relationship with the child or young person. Love could also mean handling further rejection by the young person, patiently reflecting and figuring out where both parties might have done things differently so that a way forward in the relationship can be planned. Love, around these themes, could clearly mean recognising and 'parking' our ego. 'Stickability' and unconditional acceptance are crucial.

Sometimes care workers will need to express love in ways that children and young people will not like. We may need to take decisions that are in the young person's best interests but where they perceive that their autonomy, identity, family beliefs or values are opposed. Love in this case may mean staying with the course of action or viewpoint for the right reasons. This way of loving can be expressed by workers explaining the decision-making rationale in terms of caring and respecting the young person's intrinsic human worth. This type of love will be more helpful to them than colluding with them in behaviours that will not serve them well, or worse – that mean that they are physically or emotionally unsafe.

Workers must reflect on whose needs are being met in their relationships with individual young people and where surface-level expressions of love need to be managed in the context of different presentations of attachment behaviours. 'Fluffy' love that does not hold young people accountable for their actions is not helpful. Dilemmas that require awkward and deeply sensitive decisions are a necessary part of the emotional labour required of loving workers and caregivers. Sustaining a robust loving culture cannot be complete without workers' regular discussions about their psychological and emotional limits and how these are communicated to young people in a way that does not shame them. Self-awareness is key and love must be trauma sensitive even though this is difficult and uncomfortable.

We also need to be careful of the messages caregivers receive about their own roles when they are trying to develop a culture of love in the care system. If a care worker does not love the children in the same way as a colleague, is their love less? Is their competency in their role reduced? Or is their love enough, because they made every effort within their own capacity and emotional reserves? It would undermine the quality of care received if caregivers, who may already be experiencing vicarious trauma, thought that they had failed in some way because they didn't love enough. Loving children in care is a tricky balance of bringing your whole self to the relationship yet understanding therapeutic relational distance and protective boundaries for both the adult and child. The care sector will need to attend to this robustly at an explicit level if we are to pursue changes in norms and keep children and caregivers safe.

We also need to attend to the selection process for our care workers. Many applicants may be motivated to work in the care sector by a wish to 'right some wrongs' and offer something different than their own childhood experiences. Workers may have their own experiences of trauma that resurface in response to the presenting needs of young people they are caring for. Insight around possibly triggering themes needs to be explored for all caregivers during recruitment as a matter of course, not only for prospective foster carers. It might be helpful to consider adult attachment patterns during the selection process for residential childcare. Investment at the recruitment stage will work towards cultures of safe and loving care.

In addition, we need a strong focus on talent management and clear strategies to retain caregivers who are skilled and confident in co-regulation and loving children. Part of a sound retention strategy needs to include nurturing (and loving?) the workforce. Once a person is recruited, employers have, at the very least, a moral responsibility to support their emotional well-being and development. By taking this seriously, the employer paves the way for workers' potential for loving children to flourish. Lucky is the caregiver who feels emotionally contained, acknowledged and heard by their supervisors; and who can bring their vulnerabilities to supervision, secure in the expectation that issues arising will be explored in a supportive way.

Validation of supervisees' feelings is not difficult and does not cost any money. However, it requires application of emotional intelligence and a supervisor who is self-aware and self-regulated before applying any technical expertise to the work. Our children need their caregivers to receive reflective, asset-based supervision as the norm to increase their capacity for practising in loving ways. Shame-based and tick-box supervision does not cut it.

To generate and sustain loving human systems in our residential care homes, supervisors must also acutely realise and name the exhausting paradox for carers where children experience emotional pain through healing and growth in their relational capacity. This is around the subtle, intense and sometimes explosive ways children go about engineering rejection by caregivers when they sense relationships strengthening. This 'love paradox' for children in care needs to be discussed openly and specifically with care workers in supervision. The supervisor must also sincerely work to understand the difference (and relationship) between exhaustion and compassion fatigue, and the impact this will have on the workers' capacity to love. For love to permeate through the system, workers need their managers to value and promote self-care – to understand the meanings and limitations to this in residential childcare where complex human systems, as discussed previously, always teeter on the edge of chaos.

So, we need to carefully think about methods and measures of recruiting people with the right mix of skills and values into crucial first-line supervisory roles. We must fully consider succession planning strategies to grow leaders in residential childcare who understand how to manage and support a loving culture. Our children need leaders who practise kindness every day.

## Can we put love on the agenda in supervision?

**Can we set aside time for deep reflection on love?**

**How do we plan to support people within these conversations?**

## Some reflective questions for the agenda

What did love look like in our house today? And why does this matter?

What did love feel like in our house today? Where was it good and where was it difficult?

How do you manage the sense of responsibility if you decide to say that you love individual children?

If we do decide to say we love a child, when is the right time and place for them and for us?

When are the times when feeling and acting on love is more important than saying the word 'love'?

How do we understand the early years experiences of this young person? What is our evidence of this, and how do we make sense of how to approach the love they now need?

How have any traumatic relational experiences impacted on this child's capacity to give and receive love?

What does this child understand about love?

What impact is the child's presentation of love having on you?

What extra reading on attachment do we need to seek out?

What impact is your love having on the child?

Where are we uncomfortable with love in this care setting?

Where is there confusion over what love is for the children here?

Where do we need to do some more reflection over the meaning of love for individual children and individual workers' relationships with children?

Where are workers differing in their assessment and values around loving children?

What feedback are you receiving from fellow workers about how you are practising with love?

What is your definition of the boundaries that you are putting in place to help keep you and the young person psychologically safe?

Where have boundaries been overstepped and what have you done about this?

How do we prepare to understand the complex ways in which the young person might be worried and pleased at the same time to feel loved?

How do you show love when the young person behaves in ways you do not approve of? And how do you manage your own anxiety and self-regulation?

Where have you experienced a rupture in your relationship with a young person and how have you approached your role in repairing this?

What would make a difference in helping our young people to experience safe love here?

What would you do differently if you could start again with this child?

What do you need from a supervisor to support your relationship with this child or young person?

# THE EARNED WISDOM OF CHILDREN

I thought of asking for comment and suggestions on good childcare practice from some children and young people who have earned wisdom from living in residential childcare. I quickly realised that their feedback, although crucially important, would reflect the perspective of those individuals only, and in that specific time, space and place.

Instead, I want to offer a brief format for what agencies might wish to ask children and young people in their service contexts. This action research may help policy and practice development in individual care settings.

The following are suggestions for possible research questions (supported by staff with whom the young people have a trusting relationship).

| Question 1 | What has been the best decision a worker has made for you (or with you) here? |
| Question 2 | What decisions are good workers uncomfortable with here? |
| Question 3 | What do the workers do well as a staff group here? |
| Question 4 | Can you give examples of when workers have been kind to you? |
| Question 5 | Can you give examples of when workers have been fair with you? |
| Question 6 | When you have had a disagreement with a worker, what have they done well to get your relationship back on track? |
| Question 7 | What do you think workers need to know before they get a job here? |
| Question 8 | What do you think the people in charge need to know about workers before they give them a job? |
| Question 9 | If you were a worker here, what decisions would you make differently? |
| Question 10 | If you woke up one morning and a miracle had happened in the night – this was a perfect residential house – what would it look like, and what would the workers do perfectly? |

*How will you adapt the questions to suit the developmental stages of the children you care for?*

*How will you ensure the impartiality and objectivity of this research?*

*How will you use the feedback from young people in training sessions, training programmes and debriefs?*

The following are some reflective questions around co-production with children and young people.

• Do we need a structure or strategy for co-production?

• Does the structure or strategy need to change for different purposes?

- What will our ethos of participation consist of?

- How will we capture feedback presented in inopportune ways?

- How will confidentiality be handled?

- How can we tell children and young people what their contribution in co-production will mean? What will be expected of them and what can they expect in return?

- How can we make the subject matter engaging?

- How will we ensure the language is always accessible?

- How can we make participation in policy change meaningful?

- Where is an end goal unnecessary?

- How can the quieter voices be heard?

- How and where will we record the contributions and who has made them?

- How will individual contributions be celebrated or protected from negative recourse?

- How can we be honest and how can we communicate this?

- How will the children and young people know they have been successful in meaningful co-production?

- Where can young people's leadership skills be enhanced?

- How will the appropriate boundaries of final decision making be communicated?

- Have young people got a seat at the adult decision-making table?

- When the children's feedback results in changes, how can we tell them and thank them?

- If a young person has moved on by the time a key decision is made, what will be our position on contacting them to let them know the outcome of their contribution?

## Notes

A culture of participation and joint decision making is much more meaningful and effective than a single activity in isolation.

We don't need extra funding to listen to and respect the views of people with earned wisdom.

# END NOTES

The children I have invented for these case studies are far more colourful in my imagination than I am able to represent in these few pages. Although they are of course not based on anyone I know, I felt I did get to know them as I wrote, and I became invested in their fictional care. I was reminded again what a unique privilege it is to work in the life-space and that recovery and change are possible.

The responses to the situations outlined in the stories might have turned out differently in real-time practice for you and your teams. These notes don't necessarily suggest my own judgement or provide a 'how to' guide, but I hope they offer material for reflection. I hope you can challenge the decision making in the case studies in your team discussions and that the children and young people in your care benefit from your learning.

For people entering the field of residential childcare for the first time, I hope you will be made welcome and that you are ready to meet the challenge.

If you would like to read more, the following titles may be helpful.

## Further reading

Archer, C, Drury, C and Hills, J (2015) *Healing the Hidden Hurts*. London: Jessica Kingsley Publishing.

Bomber, L (2020) *Know Me to Teach Me*. Belper: Worth Publishing.

Brierley, A (2021) *Connecting with Young People in Trouble*. Reading: Waterside Press.

Cameron, C and Moss, P (2011) *Social Pedagogy and Working with Children and Young People: Where Care and Education Meet*. London: Jessica Kingsley Publishing.

Harris, A (2012) *I'm Ok, You're Ok: A Practical Guide to Transactional Analysis*. London: Arrow.

Hughes, D (2009) *Principles of Attachment Focused Parenting: Effective Strategies to Care for Children*. New York: W W Norton & Co.

Hughes, D (2012) *Emotional and Behavioural Difficulties*. London: CoramBAAF.

Hughes, D (2017) *Building the Bonds of Attachment: Awakening Love in Deeply Traumatized Children*. Washington: Rowman & Littlefield Publishers.

Hughes, D and Baylin, J (2012) *Brain-Based Parenting*. New York: W W Norton & Co.

Hughes, D and Baylin, J (2016) *The Neurobiology of Attachment-Focused Parenting*. New York: W W Norton & Co.

Mate, G (2015) *In the Realm of Hungry Ghosts*. London: Vermillion.

Perry, A (ed) (2009) *Teenagers and Attachment*. Belper: Worth Publishing.

Perry, B (2017) *The Boy Who Was Raised as a Dog*. New York: Basic Books.

Rothschild, B (2010) *8 Keys to Safe Trauma Recovery*. New York: W W Norton & Co.

Seigel, D (2011) *Mindsight*. London: One World.

Seigel, D and Payne-Bryson, T (2012) *The Whole Brain Child: 12 Proven Strategies to Nurture Your Child's Developing Mind*: Los Gatos, CA: Robinson.

Smith, M, Fulcher, L and Doran, P (2013) *Residential Childcare in Practice: Making a Difference*. Bristol: Policy Press.

Sunderland, M (2015) *Conversations That Matter: Talking with Children and Teenagers in Ways That Help*. Belper: Worth Publishing.

Trieschman, A and Whittaker, J (2017) *The Other 23 Hours: Child Care Work with Emotionally Disturbed Children in a Therapeutic Milieu*. London: Routledge.

# THEORY TO INFORM RESIDENTIAL CHILDCARE PRACTICE

*Note: This list is indicative and aimed to prompt further reading and critical reflection.*

| Theory | Accountability |
|--------|----------------|
| Theorist | Lerner and Tetlock (1999) |

Accountability is the awareness, evaluation and accepting of responsibility.

The widely used ladder of accountability (albeit anonymous) followed Lerner and Tetlock's (1999) work.

| | |
|--------|--------|
| Accountable behaviours (Things happen because of you) | I make it happen |
| | I seek solutions |
| | I own it |
| | I acknowledge reality |
| Victim behaviours (Things happen to you) | I wait and hope |
| | I make excuses |
| | I blame and complain |
| | I am unaware/unconscious |

| Theory | Assumptive world |
|--------|------------------|
| Theorist | Kauffman (2002) |

Our assumptive world is the beliefs that ground us and make us feel secure, the beliefs that give us meaning and purpose. We are psychologically unprepared for the trauma of losing this 'world' because it is good and safe. The loss of this familiarity places one's sense of identity at risk.

*'I didn't think it would happen to me.'*

| Theory | Attachment |
|---|---|
| Theorist | Bowlby (1979); Ainsworth and Bell (1970) (strange situation); Main (1977) (disorganised attachment categorisation) |

Young children need to develop a relationship with at least one caregiver for normal social and emotional development. This can be evidenced by the child proximity seeking an attachment figure in stressful situations.

• *Secure attachment*: child explores freely when caregiver is present; child is upset when caregiver departs and happy to see caregiver return. Attentive caregivers result in children who are more prone to secure attachment patterns.

• *Anxious-ambivalent*: child will explore little, wary of strangers even when caregiver is present. When caregiver departs, child is highly distressed. Child ambivalent when caregiver returns.

• *Anxious-avoidant*: child ignores caregiver, showing little emotion when caregiver leaves/returns. The infants' needs are not met frequently, and the child may have come to believe that they have no impact on caregivers. They do not expect that their needs will be met.

• *Disorganised attachment*: child displays disorientated behaviours towards caregiver, not fitting any pattern. This may be in response to a caregiver who is themselves frightened, or who the child perceives to be frightening.

| Theory | Bereavement (grief) |
|---|---|
| Theorist | Kübler-Ross (1969); Boss (2009); Doka (1989) |

**Kübler-Ross (1969)**

The loss of a loved one who has died is the most commonly recognised form of bereavement, although the sense of grief can be felt with other losses.

**Kübler-Ross's five stages are:**

1. denial;

2. anger;

3. bargaining;

4. depression;

5. acceptance.

**Boss (2009)**

Complex and ambiguous grief occurs when a loved one is physically present but psychologically absent. Dementia is one example; psychologically absent parenting is another. Closure for those experiencing complex and ambiguous grief is difficult to resolve.

**Doka (1989)**

Disenfranchised grief refers to any grief that goes unacknowledged or unvalidated by social norms. This kind of grief is often minimised or not understood by others, which makes it particularly hard to process and work through. Examples of where this might occur are death through abortion, miscarriage, death of a partner who had had an extra-marital affair or death by socially stigmatised reasons, like addiction or suicide. Loss of a child by adoption or loss of a family member who has been unknown to the person may bring this type of stigmatised grieving.

| Theory | Classical conditioning |
|--------|------------------------|
| Theorist | Pavlov (1927) |

Behaviourist theory – Pavlov noticed that dogs would salivate before food was given to them, in response to environmental cues that the food was coming. For humans, this theory also bears out – classical conditioning is when one stimulus paired with another stimulus produces a response, thus conditioning the person to behave in a certain way.

| Theory | Cognition |
|--------|-----------|
| Theorist | Piaget (1995) |

**The sensorimotor stage (birth to two years)**

Major characteristics and development changes:

• the infant knows the world through their movements and sensations;

• children learn about the world through basic actions such as sucking, grasping, looking and listening;

• infants learn that things continue to exist even though they cannot be seen (object permanence);

• they realise that their actions can cause things to happen in the world around them.

**The pre-operational stage (ages two to seven)**

Major characteristics and development changes:

• children begin to think symbolically and learn to use words and pictures to represent objects;

• children at this stage tend to be egocentric and struggle to see things from the perspective of others;

• while they are getting better with language and thinking, they still tend to think about things in very concrete terms.

**The concrete operational stage (ages seven to eleven)**

Major characteristics and development changes:

• children begin to think logically about concrete events;

• children begin to understand the concept of conservation (for example, that the amount of liquid in a short, wide cup is equal to that in a tall, skinny glass);

• their thinking becomes more logical and organised, but still very concrete;

• children begin using inductive logic or reasoning from specific information to a general principle.

**The formal operational stage (ages 12 and up)**

Major characteristics and development changes:

• the adolescent or young adult begins to think abstractly and can reason about hypothetical problems – the ability to think about abstract ideas and situations is the key hallmark of the formal operational stage of development;

• teens begin to think more about moral, philosophical, ethical, social and political issues that require theoretical and abstract reasoning;

• they begin to use deductive logic or reasoning from a general principle to specific information;

• at this point people become capable of seeing multiple potential solutions to problems and think more scientifically about the world around them;

• systematically planning for the future: using reasoning about hypothetical situations is also a critical ability that emerges during this stage.

| Theory | Complexity |
|---|---|
| Theorist | Furnivall (2018); for the origins of complexity theory please research further. |

Connected to systems theory but much wider, taking into account influences from outside the core system. In the case of residential childcare this could mean influences of legislation, policy, characteristics of the sector, language used, location of the service, self-organising hierarchies, sustaining or counter-productive practices or historic behaviour of the system. All elements interact dynamically whereby small influences can cause large effects. Differing from systems theory, the overall behaviour of the complex system is not predicted by the behaviour of the individual elements. It can be difficult to define boundaries of complex systems. It is thought that complex systems are always on the edge of chaos.

| Theory | Crisis |
|--------|--------|
| Theorist | Roberts (1991) |

Crisis can be defined as when a person reaches the end of their coping capacity. What one person deems as a crisis may not be the same as the next person because everyone has a different level of resilience, worldview and perception of self-efficacy.

Roberts' (1991) model of crisis intervention is as follows.

1. Plan and conduct a thorough biopsychosocial and lethality/imminent danger assessment.

2. Make psychological contact and rapidly establish the collaborative relationship.

3. Identify the major problems, including crisis precipitants.

4. Encourage an exploration of feelings and emotions.

5. Generate and explore alternatives and new coping strategies.

6. Restore functioning through implementation of an action plan.

7. Plan follow-up and booster sessions.

| Theory | Drama triangle |
|--------|----------------|
| Theorist | Karpman (1968) |

This theory is a key part of transactional analysis and comprises three roles: persecutor, rescuer and victim.

The victim is not an actual victim but assumes this role. They appear helpless and find it difficult to solve problems. The persecutor appears controlling, critical, angry, authoritative and superior. The rescuer needs to be needed and enables the victim to remain dependent and gives them permission to fail.

We shift roles around the drama as situations unfold. We need to recognise where the triangle is at play and become neutral to step away from the drama and change the interactions.

| Theory | Emotional intelligence |
|--------|------------------------|
| Theorist | Goleman (1996) |

Emotional intelligence is the ability to understand, use and manage your own emotions to relieve stress, communicate effectively, overcome challenges and defuse conflict.

The five components are self-awareness, self-regulation, social skills, motivation and empathy.


| Theory | Group dynamics |
|--------|----------------|
| Theorist | Tuckman (1965); Kormanski and Mozenter (1987) |

Tuckman believed that there were four stages of group development.

1. Forming: people are anxious, curious, getting used to each other.

2. Storming: people start to push against established boundaries. Conflict arises and authority is challenged.

3. Norming: people start to resolve differences and appreciate each other's strengths – they are more comfortable asking for feedback and share a stronger commitment to the group.

4. Performing: the group is performing to its full potential. People work together to achieve more.

Tuckman's theory was developed further by Kormanski and Mozenter (1987), who believed that there were five stages.

| Theme | Task | Relationship outcome |
|-------|------|----------------------|
| Awareness | Commitment | Acceptance |
| Conflict | Clarification | Belonging |
| Co-operation | Involvement | Support |
| Productivity | Achievement | Pride |
| Separation | Recognition | Satisfaction |

| Theory | Human development | |
|---|---|---|
| Theorist | Erikson (1982) | |
| Birth to 1 year | Trust versus mistrust | Trust in primary caregiver and in one's own ability to make things happen (secure attachment to caregiver is key). |
| Age 1–5 | Autonomy versus shame and doubt | Will: new physical skills lead to demand for more choices, most often seen as saying 'no' to caregivers; child learns self-care skills such as toileting. |
| Age 3–6 | Initiative versus guilt | Purpose: ability to organise activities around some goal; more assertiveness and aggressiveness. |
| Age 6–12 | Industry versus inferiority | Competence: cultural skills and norms, including school skills and tool use (failure to master these leads to a sense of inferiority). |
| Age 12–18 | Identity versus role confusion | Fidelity: adaption of sense of self to pubertal changes; consideration of future choices, achievement of a more mature sexual identity and search for new values. |
| Age 18–30 | Intimacy versus isolation | Love: person develops intimate relationships beyond adolescent love; many become parents. |
| Age 30 – late adulthood | Generativity versus stagnation | Care: people rear children, focus on occupational achievement or creativity, and train the next generation; turn outward from the self towards others. |
| Late adulthood | Integrity versus despair | Wisdom: person conducts a life review, integrates earlier stages and comes to terms with basic identity; develops self-acceptance. |

Table reproduced from Boyd and Bee (2009)

| Theory | Identity |
|---|---|
| Theorist | Goffman (1992) |
| Goffman believed that when we are born, we are thrust onto a stage called everyday life, and that our socialisation consists of learning how to play our assigned roles from other people. We enact our roles in the company of others, who are in turn enacting their roles in interaction with us. He believed that whatever we do, we are playing out some role on the stage of life. | |

| Theory | Labelling |
|---|---|
| Theorist | Becker (1963) |
| Social groups create deviance by making rules where there are lines between those who comply with the norm and those who do not. Deviants are 'labelled' as outsiders. | |

| Theory | Learned helplessness |
|---|---|
| Theorist | Maier and Seligman (1976) |
| People believe that success and failure is independent of their own skilled actions and have difficulty perceiving that their own skilled responses are effective. | |

| Theory | Learning styles |
|---|---|
| Theorist | Barbe et al (1979); Honey and Mumford (2006) |

**Barbe et al – VAK**

People fit into one predominant model, either:

• visualising modality;

• auditory modality;

• kinesthetic modality.

This theory has been criticised as trivial and superficial.

**Honey and Mumford – learning styles**

Adapted from Kolb's experiential learning model, they aligned the stages to:

• activist;

• reflector;

• theorist;

• pragmatist.

They assumed these styles as adaptable rather than fixed.

| Theory | Locus of control |
| --- | --- |
| Theorist | Rotter (1966) |

Locus of control refers to an individual's perception about the underlying main causes of events in their life. People with a strong internal locus of control believe that their behaviours are guided by their personal decisions and efforts, and they have control over these. Having an internal locus of control is linked to self-efficacy.

People with a strong external locus of control see their behaviours and lives as being controlled by luck, fate and other external forces. These individuals view themselves as victims where they lack power.

| Theory | Locus of evaluation |
| --- | --- |
| Theorist | Rogers (1951a) |

If a child or person is operating from an internal locus of evaluation, then they trust their own instincts and the evaluation of their actions comes from within. However, many people, and especially children, operate from an external locus of evaluation; this means they use the values of others as a guide to evaluating their own actions and ideas. Some people who have not resolved earlier development stages may look to others for approval of their actions, beliefs and judgements.

| Theory | Loss and change |
| --- | --- |
| Theorist | Parkes (1972); Marris (1974) |

Parkes (1972) suggested that there were four stages of loss and grief:

1. shock and numbness;

2. yearning and searching;

3. disorganisation and despair;

4. reorganisation and recovery.

Marris (1974) considered that loss and grief could be brought about from loss of structures of meaning – so people can experience loss from aspects wider than bereavement, for example, places, predictable social contexts or identity. Changes in life, even positive, yearned-for changes, can prompt a sense of loss. For example, having a baby also means loss of a 'carefree' lifestyle.

| Theory | Mastery |
|---|---|
| Theorist | Bloom (1981) |

Mastery learning maintains that students must achieve a level of mastery in prerequisite knowledge before moving forward to learn subsequent information. The emphasis is on the support they need to accomplish mastery.

| Theory | Mentalisation |
|---|---|
| Theorist | Fonagy et al (2002) |

Mentalisation is insight into what one is feeling and why. It is thinking about what we ourselves are thinking, and what others might be thinking. It is the concept of children learning to reflect upon and understand their own states of mind. Attuning to the emotional states of others helps us anticipate how to approach different situations with people. This aspect of development can be impaired for some people due to developmental trauma.

| Theory | Moral development |
|---|---|
| Theorist | Kohlberg (1971) |

This is a six-stage theory of how humans develop into moral beings.

1. Pre-conventional morality – what authorities say is right and will accept or punish.

2. Individualism and exchange – the person is no longer impressed by any single authority. Accepts that people have different viewpoints. Punishment is a risk to be avoided. Fair exchange of deals.

3. Conventional morality – based on good interpersonal relationships. Accepts and promotes good motives based on love, empathy and trust. Can assume that this attitude will be expressed by the whole community.

4. Maintaining the social order – obeys rules. Understands that motives may be good but that anarchy will ensue if everyone broke the rules. Can elaborate on the reasoning behind the law. Can think as a fully fledged member of society.

5. Social contracts and individual rights – can think about society in a theoretical way. Considers rights and values that a society ought to uphold. Can evaluate existing societies in terms of these prior considerations. Values democratic procedures.

6. Universal principles – the person will not vote for a law which aids some but hinders others. Believes in equal rights and true justice.

| Theory | Motivation |
|---|---|
| Theorist | Deci (1971); deCharms (1968) |

Motivation is a desire or drive to act. Motivation can either be intrinsic (arising from internal factors) or extrinsic (arising from external factors).

Intrinsically motivated behaviours are performed because of the sense of personal satisfaction that they bring (Deci, 1971).

Extrinsically motivated behaviours are performed in order to receive something from others or to avoid negative outcomes. Extrinsic rewards could be sweets, a sticker, a job promotion, praise and recognition (deCharms, 1968).

Also see hierarchy of needs/motivation (Maslow, 1943).


| Theory | Multiple intelligences |
|---|---|
| Theorist | Gardner (1983) |

Gardner believed that we are not born with all the intelligence that we are capable of and that our abilities are more than a general intelligence. He proposed that these are:

1. musical, rhythmic and harmonic;

2. visual-spatial;

3. linguistic verbal;

4. logical-mathematical;

5. bodily-kinaesthetic;

6. interpersonal;

7. intrapersonal;

8. naturalistic (added by Gardner in 1995);

9. existential (added by Gardner in 1999).

| Theory | Need |
|---|---|
| Theorist | Maslow (1943); Bradshaw (1972) |

Maslow's hierarchy of needs

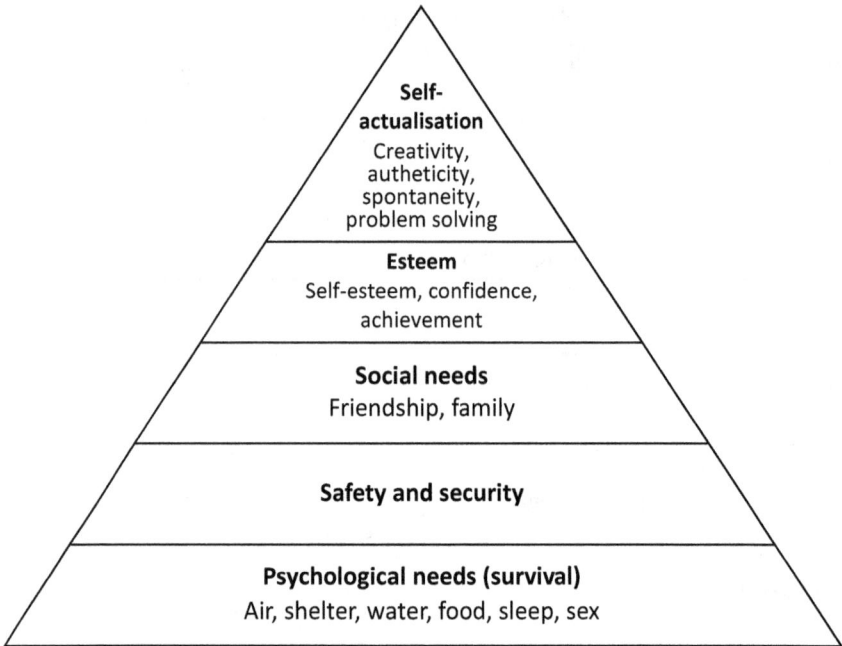

| Bradshaw's Taxonomy of Need | |
|---|---|
| Normative need | Based on professional judgement – eg need for treatment |
| Felt need | Individuals' perceptions of variations from normal health (and well-being) |
| Expressed need | Vocalisation of need/how people use services |
| Comparative need | Based on professional judgement as to the needs of different groups |

| Theory | Neurosequential model |
|--------|----------------------|
| Theorist | Perry (2011) |

This is how the brain develops.

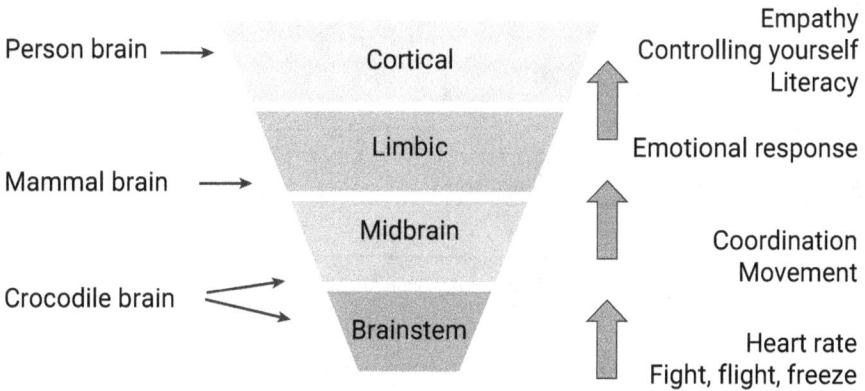

Perry's neurosequential model:

- Person brain → Cortical — Empathy, Controlling yourself, Literacy
- Limbic — Emotional response
- Mammal brain → Midbrain — Coordination, Movement
- Crocodile brain → Brainstem — Heart rate, Fight, flight, freeze

Perry's neurosequential model, after Perry (2011)

This indicates that we need to respond to young people with the following model.

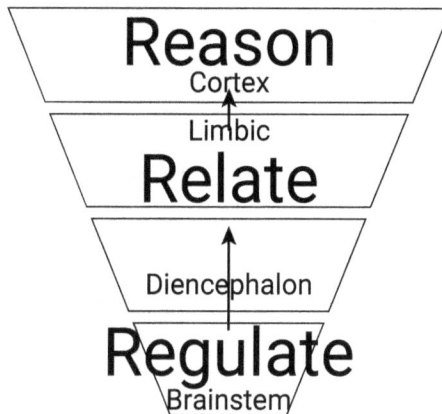

Sequence of engagement:

- Reason — Cortex
- Limbic — Relate
- Diencephalon
- Regulate — Brainstem

Sequence of engagement, after Perry (2011)

This is especially important where the effects of trauma on young people mean that they are easily triggered and can behave from the 'feelings' part rather than their 'thinking' part of their brain.

| Theory | Operant conditioning |
| --- | --- |
| Theorist | Skinner (1950) |

Behaviourist theory – Skinner saw the learner as more active than Pavlov did. He saw behaviour as being shaped by positive or negative reinforcement. The ABC of behaviour is:

- **A**ntecedent;

- **B**ehaviour;

- **C**onsequence.

| Theory | Planned behaviour (intention) |
| --- | --- |
| Theorist | Azjen (1991) |

People make logical, reasoned decisions to engage in specific behaviours by evaluating the information available to them.

So, the likelihood of a person engaging in a behaviour is correlated with the strength of their intention to engage in the behaviour. Factors influencing this include the person's attitude to towards the behaviour, the person's perception of group norms concerning the behaviour and the extent to which the person perceives that they have control over the behaviour.

(Also linked to self-efficacy.)

| Theory | Power |
| --- | --- |
| Theorist | French and Raven (1959) |

Five bases of power.

1. *Legitimate*: this comes from the belief that a person has the formal right to make demands, and to expect others to be compliant and obedient.

2. *Reward*: this results out of one person's ability to compensate another for compliance.

3. *Expert*: this is based on a person's high levels of skill and knowledge.

4. *Referent*: this is the result of a person's perceived attractiveness, worthiness and right to others' respect.

5. *Coercive*: this comes from the belief that a person can punish others for non-compliance.

Six years later, Raven (1965) added an extra power base.

6. *Informational*: This comes from a person's ability to control the information that others need to accomplish something.

By understanding these different forms of power, we can learn to use the positive ones to full effect and be alert to situations where people are disempowered.

| Theory | Rational choice |
|---|---|
| Theorist | Cornish and Clarke (1986) |

People weigh up means and ends, costs and benefits before making a choice. These choices are always framed through our worldview.

| Theory | Resilience |
|---|---|
| Theorist | Rutter (1985); Gilligan (1998) |

**Rutter (1985)**

Resilience is positive adaptation after a stressful or adverse situation. Different people can apparently cope with different amounts of stress and vary in their ability to navigate the life course with competent functioning. Protective factors such as housing stability, good health, freedom from poverty and violence, and supportive relationships promote resilience.

**Gilligan (1998)**

The degree of resilience demonstrated by a person in the adverse context may be related to the extent to which that context has elements that nurture resilience. Supportive relationships are key.

| Theory | Self-efficacy |
|---|---|
| Theorist | Bandura and Adams (1977) |

Perceived self-efficacy affects people's choice of activities and behavioural settings, how much effort they expend, and how long they will persist in the face of obstacles and aversive experiences. The stronger the perceived self-efficacy, the more active the coping efforts.

Those who persist in subjectively threatening activities will eventually eliminate their inhibitions through corrective experience, whereas those who avoid what they fear or who cease their coping efforts prematurely will retain their self-debilitating expectations and defensive behaviour.

| Theory | Social constructionism |
|---|---|
| Theorist | Bannister and Mair (1968) |

This is the idea that everything is socially constructed and there is no universal acceptance of truth. Reality is dependent upon which lens we are viewing the world through. We need to consider how we construct the narrative, our own and that of others. We need to pay attention to how use of language contributes to this in negative or stigmatising ways, and what we can do to promote anti-oppressive narratives.

| Theory | Social learning theory |
|--------|------------------------|
| Theorist | Bandura (1977) |
| Social learning is when we copy other people's behaviour. We learn by following the behaviour of role models. The most famous experiment is the 'Bobo doll' conducted by Albert Bandura (1977). | |

| Theory | Social pedagogy |
|--------|-----------------|
| Theorist | Hämäläinen (2003) |
| Associated with German and Scandinavian traditions; social pedagogy validates the learning in everyday life-space activities, especially those that involve negotiation and co-production. Activities are regarded as 'the common third' and are where care and education meet. This model encompasses strengths-based practice where risk is considered necessary for growth. See also https://beaconhouse.org.uk/resources | |

| Theory | Stigma |
|--------|--------|
| Theorist | Goffman (1963) |
| A social stigma is an attribute, behaviour or reputation which is socially discrediting in a particular way. It causes an individual to be mentally classified by others in an undesirable, rejected stereotype rather than be accepted. | |

| Theory | Stress vulnerability |
|--------|----------------------|
| Theorist | Zubin and Spring (1977) |
| People with low vulnerability need to experience a great deal of stress before they become distressed. People with a high level of vulnerability need only a small amount of stress before they become unwell. Stress leads first to anxiety and then, if not understood and checked, this anxiety can tip the person into a mental health crisis. | |

| Theory | Systems |
|---|---|
| Theorist | Parsons (1975) |

A system is a group of inter-related, interdependent parts and can be natural or manufactured. Every system has boundaries and is defined by structure and purpose. It can intertwine with other systems and have many influencing contexts. A system is more than the sum of its parts. Changing one part of the system may affect other parts or the whole system. It may be possible to predict changes in systems.

| Theory | Transactional analysis |
|---|---|
| Theorist | Berne (1964) |

This theory of communication is a means of examining the transactions between people. Berne (1964) said that people are all made up of three ego states: Parent, Child and Adult. Both the giver and receiver of communication transactions act in one of the ego states. Successful transactions will be complementary. They must go back from the receiving ego state to the sending ego state. For example, if the stimulus is Parent to Child, the response must be Child to Parent, or the transaction will be 'crossed' and there will be a problem between the sender and receiver.

If a crossed transaction occurs, there is ineffective communication. Worse still, either or both parties will be upset. In order for the relationship to continue smoothly, the agent or respondent must remedy the situation with a complementary transaction.

| Theory | Transitions |
|---|---|
| Theorist | Bridges (1995) |

• Endings: letting go and managing the loss of what will be no longer.

• Neutral zone: lost between the old and the new. A messy place where anything could happen. Psychological realignment starts to take place.

• New beginnings: new identities and values emerge. Energy returns.

Morale dips in the neutral zone and picks up again with new beginnings.

| Theory | Trauma |
|---|---|
| Theorist | Suggested further research by writers such as Bruce Perry, Peter Levine, Bessel Van der Kolk, Stephen Porges and Gabor Mate (please seek out these and other researchers). |

Trauma is the response to a deeply distressing or disturbing experience that overwhelms the individual's ability to cope. This can be a single event or a course of experiences lasting a number of years. It causes feelings of helplessness and diminishes the person's sense of self and self-efficacy, and their ability to feel a full range of emotions. The timing of the trauma is significant in the person's development.

| Theory | Unconditional positive regard |
|---|---|
| Theorist | Rogers (1951b) |

Unconditional positive regard is the basic acceptance and support of a person regardless of what the person says or does. It is used as a foundation for working with people and underpins the humanistic approach.

# References

Ainsworth, M D and Bell, S M (1970) Attachment, Exploration, and Separation: Illustrated by the Behavior of One-Year-Olds in a Strange Situation. *Child Development*, 41(1): 49–67.

Azjen, I (1991) The Theory of Planned Behavior. *Organizational Behavior and Human Decision Processes*, 50(2): 179–211

Bandura, A (1977) *Social Learning Theory*. Englewood Cliffs, NJ: Prentice Hall.

Bandura, A and Adams, N E (1977) Analysis of Self-efficacy Theory of Behavioural Change. *Cognitive Therapy and Research*, 1(4): 287–310.

Bannister, D and Mair, J M (1968) *The Evaluation of Personal Constructs*. London: Academic Press.

Barbe, W B, Swassing, R H and Milone, M N (1979). *Teaching Through Modality Strengths: Concepts and Practices*. Columbus, OH: Zaner-Bloser.

Becker, H (1963) *Outsiders*. New York: Free Press.

Berne, E (1964) *Games People Play*. New York: Ballantine Books.

Bloom, B S (1981) *All Our Children Learning: A Primer for Parents, Teachers, and Other Educators*. London: McGraw-Hill.

Boss, P (2009) The Trauma and Complicated Grief of Ambiguous Loss. *Pastoral Psychology*, 59: 137–45.

Bowlby, J (1979) *The Making and Breaking of Affectional Bonds*. London: Routledge.

Boyd, D and Bee, H (2009) *Lifespan Development*. Boston, MA: Pearson Education, Inc.

Bradshaw, J (1972) Taxonomy of Social Need. In McLachlan, G (ed) *Problems and Progress in Medical Care: Essays on Current Research* (7th series, pp 71–82). London: Oxford University Press.

Bridges, W (1995) *Managing Transitions: Making the Most of Change*. London: Nicholas Brierley Publishing.

Cornish, D and Clarke, R V (eds) (1986). Introduction. In Cornish, D and Clarke, R V (eds) *The Reasoning Criminal*. New York: Springer-Verlag.

DeCharms, R (1968) *Personal Causation*. New York: Academic Press.

Deci, E (1971) Effects of Externally Mediated Rewards on Intrinsic Motivation. *Journal of Personality and Social Psychology*, 18(1): 105–15.

Doka, K (ed) (1989) *Disenfranchised Grief: Recognizing Hidden Sorrow*. Lexington, MA: Lexington Books.

Erikson, E H (1982) *The Lifecycle Completed*. New York: W W Norton.

Fonagy, P, Gergely, G, Jurist, E and Target, M (2002). *Affect Regulation, Mentalization and the Development of the Self*. New York: Other Press.

French, J R P and Raven, B (1959) The Bases of Social Power. In D P Cartwright (ed) *Studies in Social Power* (pp 259–69). Ann Arbor, MI: Institute for Social Research, University of Michigan.

Furnivall, J (2018) Reclaiming Complexity: Beneath the Surface in Residential Childcare. *Journal of Social Work Practice*, 34(4): 373–90.

Gardner, H (1983) *Frames of Mind: The Theory of Multiple Intelligences*. London: Fontana Press.

Gilligan, R (1998) The Importance of Schools and Teachers in Child Welfare. *Child & Family Social Work*, 3(1): 13–26.

Goffman, E (1963) *Stigma: Notes on the Management of a Spoiled Identity*. New York: Simon & Schuster.

Goffman, E (1992) *The Presentation of Self in Everyday Life*. London: Penguin.

Goleman, D (1996) *Emotional Intelligence: Why It Can Matter More Than IQ*. London: Bloomsbury.

Hämäläinen J (2003) The Concept of Social Pedagogy in the Field of Social Work. *Journal of Social Work*, 3(1): 69–80.

Honey, P and Mumford, A (2006) *Learning Styles Questionnaire: 80-Item Version*. Maidenhead: Peter Honey Publications.

Karpman, S (1968) Fairy Tales and Script Drama Analysis. *Transactional Analysis Bulletin*, 26(7): 39–43.

Kauffman, J (2002) *Loss of the Assumptive World: A Theory of Traumatic Loss*. London: Brunner-Routledge.

Kohlberg, L (1971) From 'Is' to 'Ought': How to Commit the Naturalistic Fallacy and Get Away with It in the Study of Moral Development. In Mischel, T (ed) *Cognitive Development and Epistemology* (pp 91–107). New York: Academic Press.

Kormanski, C and Mozenter, A (1987) A New Model of Team Building: A Technology for Today and Tomorrow. *The 1987 Annual: Developing Human Resources and in Theories and Models in Applied Behavioral Science, Volume 3* (p 231). San Diego: Pfeiffer Management and Leadership.

Kübler-Ross, E (1969) *On Death and Dying*. London: Routledge.

Lerner, J S and Tetlock, P E (1999) Accounting for the Effects of Accountability. *Psychological Bulletin*, 125(2): 255–75.

Maier, S F and Seligman, M E (1976) Learned Helplessness: Theory and Evidence. *Journal of Experimental Psychology: General*, 105(1): 3–46.

Main, M (1977) Analysis of a Peculiar Form of Reunion Behaviour Seen in Some Daycare Children. In Webb, R (ed) *Social Development in Childhood* (pp 33–78). Baltimore. MD: John Hopkins.

Marris, P (1974) *Loss and Change*. London: Routledge and Kegan Paul plc.

Maslow, A H (1943) A Theory of Human Motivation. *Psychological Review*, 50(4): 370–96.

Parkes, C M (1972) *Bereavement: Studies of Grief in Adult Life*. New York: International Universities Press.

Parsons, T (1975) The Present Status of 'Structural-Functional' Theory in Sociology. *Social Systems and The Evolution of Action Theory*. New York: The Free Press.

Pavlov, I P (1927) *Conditioned Reflexes*. Oxford: Oxford University Press.

Perry, B (2011) *Born for Love: Why Empathy Is Essential – and Endangered*. New York: William Morrow.

Piaget, J (1995) *Sociological Studies*. London: Routledge.

Raven, B H (1965) Social influence and power. In Steiner, D I and Fishbein, M (eds) *Current Studies in Social Psychology* (pp 371–82). New York: Holt, Rinehart, Winston.

Roberts, A R (1991) Conceptualizing Crisis Theory and the Crisis Intervention Model. In Roberts, A R (ed) *Contemporary Perspectives on Crisis Intervention and Prevention* (pp 3–17). Englewood Cliffs, NJ: Prentice Hall.

Rogers, C (1951a) *Client-Centred Therapy*. London: Constable.

Rogers, C (1951b) *Client-Centred Therapy: Its Current Practice, Implications and Theory*. Boston, MA: Houghton Mifflin.

Rotter, J B (1966) Generalised Expectancies for Internal versus External Control of Reinforcement. *Psychological Monographs: General and Applied*, 80(1): 1–28.

Rutter, M (1985) Resilience in the Face of Adversity: Protective Factors and Resistance to Psychiatric Disorder. *The British Journal of Psychiatry*, 147: 589–611.

Skinner, B F (1950) Are Theories of Learning Necessary? *Psychological Review*, 57(4): 193–216.

Tuckman, B W (1965) Developmental Sequence in Small Groups. *Psychological Bulletin*, 63(6): 384–99.

Zubin, J and Spring, B (1977) Vulnerability: A New View of Schizophrenia. *Journal of Abnormal Psychology*, 86(2): 103–26.

# INTERVENTIONS TO INFORM RESIDENTIAL CHILDCARE PRACTICE

*Note: This list is indicative to prompt further reading and critical reflection.*

| Intervention | Behaviour chain analysis |
|---|---|
| Theorist | Skinner (1938) provided the basis for this intervention and many others have used adaptations and applications of his work. |
| What is the intervention? | 1. Describe your problem behaviour.<br><br>2. Describe the specific precipitating event that triggered the chain of behaviour.<br><br>3. Describe the vulnerability factors happening before the precipitating event.<br><br>4. Describe in detail the chain of events that led up to the behaviour.<br><br>(Think about all the possible links, vulnerabilities, impacts, solutions and prevention strategies.) |

| Intervention | Cognitive behavioural therapy |
|---|---|
| Theorist | Beck and Rush (1987)<br><br>Aaron Beck is considered the forefather of cognitive behaviour therapy, but see also his more recent work with Judith Beck (Beck and Beck, 2020). |
| What is the intervention? | Cognitive behaviour therapy aims to challenge cognitive distortions and their associated behaviours to improve personal coping, emotional regulation and to solve current problems.<br><br>Cognitive distortions include:<br><br>• black and white thinking (all or nothing);<br><br>• jumping to conclusions;<br><br>• mind reading;<br><br>• fortune telling;<br><br>• labelling;<br><br>• catastrophising;<br><br>• minimising. |

| Intervention | Conflict management |
|---|---|
| Theorist | Rahim (2002)<br><br>(This is only one viewpoint so please do research other methods.) |

→

| | |
|---|---|
| What is the intervention? | Rahim noted five different management approaches to combating conflicts with an underpinning scale of 'concern for self' and 'concern for others'. These are:<br><br>1. avoiding;<br><br>2. obliging;<br><br>3. dominating;<br><br>4. integrating;<br><br>5. compromising. |

| Intervention | Co-regulation |
|---|---|
| Theorist | Based on polyvagal theory – Porges (2011) |
| What is the intervention? | Co-regulation lies at the heart of all human relationships. According to polyvagal theory, it is the reciprocal sending and receiving of signals of safety. It is not merely the absence of danger but connection between two nervous systems, each nourishing and regulating the other in the process.<br><br>This means that young people need relationships where they are emotionally nurtured. This, in turn, will help them self-regulate. |

| Intervention | Crisis intervention |
|---|---|
| Theorist | Roberts (1991) |
| What is the intervention? | Crisis can be defined as when a person reaches the end of their coping capacity. What one person deems as a crisis may not be the same as the next person because everyone has a different level of resilience, worldview and perception of self-efficacy.<br><br>Roberts' (1991) model of crisis intervention is as follows.<br><br>1. Plan and conduct a thorough biopsychosocial and lethality/imminent danger assessment.<br><br>2. Make psychological contact and rapidly establish the collaborative relationship.<br><br>3. Identify the major problems, including crisis precipitants.<br><br>4. Encourage an exploration of feelings and emotions.<br><br>5. Generate and explore alternatives and new coping strategies.<br><br>6. Restore functioning through implementation of an action plan.<br><br>7. Plan follow-up and booster sessions. |

| Intervention | De-escalation |
|---|---|
| Theorist | Bloom and Farragher (2013) |
| What is the intervention? | Communication is key. The arousal–relaxation cycle where an event triggers a young person to become physiologically aroused and possibly emotionally distressed is managed by:<br><br>• self-regulation by the adult;<br><br>• supporting the young person's self-awareness;<br><br>• co-regulation;<br><br>• validation of emotions;<br><br>• self-soothing;<br><br>• use of alternatives;<br><br>• education.<br><br>The adrenaline in the young person's body will still be present for some time after the precipitating event and support may be necessary for the young person to return to their baseline arousal state.<br><br>(Please research more about the Sanctuary Model [Bloom], which is based on trauma-sensitive practice.) |

| Intervention | Group work |
|---|---|
| Theorist | Tuckman and Jenson (1977) |
| What is the intervention? | The model is widely recognised as four stages with two more recently added:<br><br>1. storming;<br><br>2. forming;<br><br>3. norming;<br><br>4. performing;<br><br>5. mourning;<br><br>6. adjourning.<br><br>Group processes are also underpinned by systems theory and transactional analysis. Beginnings, middles and endings are a continuous part of the residential milieu as different young people join the group and then move on. Groups can also be formed for a particular focus. Workers need to attend to group processes to plan for successful experiences and outcomes for group members. |

| Intervention | Harm reduction |
|---|---|
| Theorist | Drawn from substance use fields of expertise. |
| What is the intervention? | Safe use, managed use and abstinence from substances. Harm reduction is also a movement for social justice, built on respect for the human rights of people who use substances. The ideas can be broadened out to accommodate any intervention which minimises the negative impact of illicit drug use. Harm reduction can also apply to other situations where risk reduction would be beneficial. |

| Intervention | Life-space interview |
|---|---|
| Theorist | Redl (1966) (quoted in Morris, 1991) |
| What is the intervention? | A life-space interview is a strategy which uses everyday events as an opportunity to intervene in the everyday life of a young person for therapeutic reasons. This is the model. 1. Isolate the conversation. 2. Explore the young person's point of view. 3. Summarise the feelings and the content. 4. Connect the young person's feelings and behaviours. 5. Discuss alternative behaviours. 6. Develop a plan with the young person or practise new behaviours. 7. Re-integrate the young person with the group. |

| Intervention | Life-story work |
|---|---|
| Theorist | Rose (2012) Although Richard Rose is thought of as a pioneer of the life story work model, please research other resources |
| What is the intervention? | This is the work needed to ensure that the child understands and can rationalise their situation regarding their care. For example, who they live with and why. This will include narrative about their family history. Good life-story work involves more than a 'product' – so as well as a book or memory box, the surrounding discussion (age and stage appropriate) is important. Life story work should be at the pace of the child, and professionals and carers should ensure the child has access to the available material when it is important to them. |

| Intervention | Mediation |
|---|---|
| Theorist | Dates back many thousands of years |
| What is the intervention? | Mediation is grounded in the belief that conflict offers an opportunity to build stronger individuals, more satisfying relationships and better communities. Mediation is often used to prevent the need for more formal processes to resolve conflict or dissatisfaction. |

| Intervention | Mentalisation |
|---|---|
| Theorist | Mentalisation emerged in the psychoanalytic literature in the 1960s. Fonagy (1989) is credited with application to attachment issues in human psychology. Please also see *Mindsight* by Daniel Seigel (2011) for further insights. |
| What is the intervention? | Mentalisation has been noted as 'thinking about thinking'. This is something we do all the time, to bring together an understanding of our own and others' mental states so we can anticipate and adjust our behaviours to meet our own and others' emotional needs. Mentalisation ability is weakened by intense emotion or differences in frames of reference. |

| Intervention | Mindfulness |
|---|---|
| Theorist | Mindfulness originated from ancient Eastern and Buddhist philosophy and dates back around 2500 years. The concept of mindfulness was introduced to the western world by Jon Kabat-Zinn. |
| What is the intervention? | Being mindful is the quality of being conscious or aware of something. It is also actively used as a therapeutic intervention where the person focuses awareness in the present moment while at the same time calmly acknow-ledging and accepting feelings, thoughts and sensations. |

| Intervention | Opportunity-led practice |
|---|---|
| Theorist | Ward (2002) |
| What is the intervention? | Therapeutic work is not just confined to the 'therapeutic hour'. Moments or incidents may happen during everyday care, which present chances to open up communication and insight alongside a young person. The four stages are generally observation and assessment, decision making, taking action, and closure. Residential childcare is a series of opportunities, and the skill is in the decision making of the practitioner in how to respond. This intervention is closely linked to the life-space interview. |

| Intervention | PACE |
|---|---|
| Theorist | Hughes (2009) |
| | See also Golding and Hughes (2012) |
| What is the intervention? | PACE is an acronym for: |
| | • **P**layfulness; |
| | • **A**cceptance; |
| | • **C**uriosity; |
| | • **E**mpathy. |
| | Adults who respond with PACE help build safe, trusting and meaningful relationships with children and young people who have experienced trauma. It describes a way of relating to others, or a 'way of being', paying close attention to how we deliver messages to children and young people through our communication. |

| Intervention | Relationship-based practice |
|---|---|
| Theorist | Ruch et al (2018) – this is a book recommendation, rather than a theory in itself. |
| What is the intervention? | This method of practice relies upon developing secure relationships with the person receiving a service to effect change. It is underpinned by theories of unconditional positive regard (Rogers, 1951), co-regulation (Porges, 2011), co-production (Arnstein, 1969) and emotional intelligence (Goleman, 1996). |

| Intervention | Secure base |
|---|---|
| Theorist | Schofield and Beek (2015) |
| What is the intervention? | This model promotes resilience and attachment. It provides a framework for the caregiving cycle using the dimensions of caregiving. |

| Caregiving dimension | Developmental benefit |
|---|---|
| Availability | Helping the child to trust |
| Sensitivity | Helping the child to manage feelings |
| Acceptance | Building the child's self-esteem |
| Co-operation | Helping the child to feel effective |
| Family membership | Helping the child to belong |

| Intervention | Social pedagogy |
|---|---|
| Theorist | Hämäläinen (2003) |
| What is the intervention? | Associated with German and Scandinavian traditions, social pedagogy validates the learning in everyday life-space activities, especially those that involve negotiation and co-production. Activities are regarded as 'the common third' and are where care and education meet. This model encompasses strengths-based practice where risk is considered necessary for growth. |

| Intervention | Strengths-based practice |
|---|---|
| Theorist | Multiple contributors |
| What is the intervention? | A strengths-based (or asset-based) approach explores the individual's resources, assets and characteristics in a goal-oriented way, instead of deficit-based conversations which may perpetuate the problem. |

| Intervention | Task-centred practice |
|---|---|
| Theorist | Doel and Marsh (1992) |
| What is the intervention? | Task-centred practice is a sequence of work which leads from problems to future goals and more positive outcomes.<br><br>The stages are:<br><br>1. identify the problem;<br><br>2. set goals;<br><br>3. create a plan;<br><br>4. carry out the plan;<br><br>5. evaluate the results. |

| Intervention | Trauma-sensitive practice |
|---|---|
| Theorist | Multiple contributors |
| What is the intervention? | • Listen at an appropriately attuned level.<br><br>• Create a safe and boundaried space.<br><br>• Consider what behaviour may be communicating.<br><br>• Validate the person's feelings and experiences.<br><br>• Recognise the person's core strengths.<br><br>• Offer positive affirmation of the person's values, attributes and efforts.<br><br>• Reduce barriers.<br><br>• Present choices to help the person take control for themselves.<br><br>• Help the person develop a sense of mastery.<br><br>• Be predictable.<br><br>We do not need to know the specifics of the traumatic experiences to work in this way. |

# References

Arnstein, S R (1969) A Ladder of Citizen Participation. *Journal of the American Institute of Planners*, 35(4): 216–24.

Beck, A T and Rush, A J (1987) *Cognitive Therapy of Depression*. London: Guilford Press.

Beck, J S and Beck, A T (2020) *Cognitive Behaviour Therapy: Basics and Beyond*. London: Guilford Press.

Bloom, S and Farragher, B (2013) *Restoring Sanctuary: A New Operating System for Trauma Informed Systems of Care*. Oxford: Oxford University Press.

Doel, M and Marsh, P (1992) *Task-Centred Social Work*. London: Routledge.

Fonagy, P (1989) On Tolerating Mental States: Theory of Mind in Borderline Patients. *Bulletin of the Anna Freud Centre*, 12: 91–115.

Golding, K and Hughes, D (2012) *Creating Loving Attachments: Parenting with PACE to Nurture Confidence and Security in the Troubled Child*. London: Jessica Kingsley Publishing.

Goleman, D (1996) *Emotional Intelligence: Why It Can Matter More Than IQ*. London: Bloomsbury.

Hämäläinen, J (2003) The Concept of Social Pedagogy in the Field of Social Work. *Journal of Social Work*, 3(1): 69–80.

Hughes, D (2009) *Principles of Attachment-Focused Parenting: Effective Strategies to Care for Children*. New York: W W Norton & Co.

Morris, W C (1991) *Crisis Intervention in Residential Treatment: The Clinical Innovations of Fritz Redl*. Abingdon: Routledge.

Porges, S (2011) *The Polyvagal Theory* London: W W Norton & Co.

Rahim, M A (2002) Toward a Theory of Managing Organisational Conflict. *International Journal of Conflict Management*, 13(3): 206–35.

Roberts, A R (1991) Conceptualizing Crisis Intervention and the Crisis Intervention Model. In Roberts, A R (ed) *Contemporary Perspectives on Crisis Intervention and Prevention* (pp 3–17). Englewood Cliffs, NJ: Prentice Hall.

Rogers C (1951) *Client-Centred Therapy*. London: Constable.

Rose, R (2012) *Life Story Therapy with Traumatised Children*. London: Jessica Kingsley.

Ruch, G, Turney, D, and Ward, A (eds) (2018) *Relationship-based Social Work: Getting to the Heart of Practice*. London: Jessica Kingsley Publishing.

Schofield, G and Beek, M (2015) *The Secure Base Model*. London: BAAF.

Seigel, D (2011) *Mindsight*. London: One World.

Skinner, B F (1938) *The Behavior of Organisms: An Experimental Analysis*. New York: Appleton-Century.

Tuckman, B W and Jenson, M-A C (1977) Stages of Small Group Development. *Group Organisation and Management*, 2(4): 419–27.

Ward, A (2002) Opportunity Led Work: Maximising the Possibilities for Therapeutic Communication in Everyday Interactions. *Therapeutic Communities*, 23(2): 111–24.

# INDEX

For Product Safety Concerns and Information please contact our EU
representative  GPSR@taylorandfrancis.com
Taylor & Francis Verlag GmbH, Kaufingerstraße 24, 80331 München, Germany